How To Be a Successful Radiology Practitioner Assistant/ Radiologist Assistant ©

Bhawna Oberoi, BSRS, RPA, RT (R) (M)

Practicing RPA in Dallas, Texas

TRAFFORD

Canada • USA • Spain • UK • Ireland

Note for Librarians: a cataloguing record for this book that includes Dewey Decimal Classification and US Library of Congress numbers is available from the Library and Archives of Canada. The complete cataloguing record can be obtained from their online database at:
www.collectionscanada.ca/amicus/index-e.html
ISBN 1-4120-4697-1
Printed in Victoria, BC, Canada

TRAFFORD

Offices in Canada, USA, Ireland, UK and Spain

This book was published on-demand in cooperation with Trafford Publishing. On-demand publishing is a unique process and service of making a book available for retail sale to the public taking advantage of on-demand manufacturing and Internet marketing. On-demand publishing includes promotions, retail sales, manufacturing, order fulfilment, accounting and collecting royalties on behalf of the author.

Book sales for North America and international:
Trafford Publishing, 6E–2333 Government St.,
Victoria, BC v8t 4p4 CANADA
phone 250 383 6864 (toll-free 1 888 232 4444)
fax 250 383 6804; email to orders@trafford.com

Book sales in Europe:
Trafford Publishing (uk) Ltd., Enterprise House, Wistaston Road Business Centre,
Wistaston Road, Crewe, Cheshire cw2 7rp UNITED KINGDOM
phone 01270 251 396 (local rate 0845 230 9601)
facsimile 01270 254 983; orders.uk@trafford.com
Order online at:
www.trafford.com/robots/04-2505.html

10 9 8 7 6 5 4 3

To my parents
Usha and Surendra
and
the love of my life, Tom

You have been an inspiration and a persistent tower of strength

To
RPAs, students and my friends from Weber State
who have inspired this book

Hard work is only a part of the equation, but a big part indeed

FOREWORD

An advanced practice level within radiology is an opportunity and an aspiration for all motivated technologists. For a number of years I have always felt that technologists were being utilized to their potential and were not recognized for their expansive knowledge and skills. A contributing reason for not being recognized for their talents is the willingness of technologists to absorb tasks and responsibilities, without compensation or vertical mobility. In observing other mid-level health professionals functioning in medical imaging, it was obvious that performing at an advanced practice level within the field was a natural niche for technologists.

The opportunity for development of a mid-level health professional in radiology came when Weber State University was approached in 1994 by the Department of Defense to develop a program preparing the technologist to assume a role as a primary health care provider in radiology services. Although the Department of Defense could not follow through due to budget restraints, the program had been developed and technologists were eager to enroll. The first class was admitted in 1996 with ten students participating. As knowledge of the program spread and as students and graduates became successful in the clinical area, the major organizations became interested and have attempted to shape this advanced practice level. However, the role had been cast, with technologists certified as Radiology Practitioner Assistants (RPAs) forging in-roads with organizations and state and federal entities. The RPAs have been courageous in the pursuit of recognition of this advanced practice level for medical imaging and in assisting technologists gain recognition for their capabilities and abilities.

The book answers may questions applicants and students have when applying to either a RPA or a RA program. Especially important are the methods used to gain confidence and to establish relationships in clinical areas. The information is also especially helpful in creating an awareness of what to expect and what the expectations are, in regard to functioning as an RPA/RA student. It has been a pleasure for me to write a foreword to this book because it will be an indispensable tool for anyone contemplating a career move to a mid-level healthcare provider in radiology.

Jane Van Valkenburg, PhD RT (R) (N), FASRT
Educational Director and Professor
Radiology Practitioner Assistant Program
Weber State University
Ogden, Utah

FOREWORD

This handbook was written by Bhawna Oberoi, who is a Registered Radiologic Technologist with several years of experience prior to her completion of the Radiology Practitioner Assistant Advance Degree Program, Department of Radiologic Sciences, Weber State University, Ogden, Utah.

Her intended purpose was to inform other technologists and radiologists about the newest profession in radiology—Radiology Practitioner Assistant (RPA) with references to the Radiology Assistant (RA), which is a derivative of the RPA, for experienced registered radiographers and radiologists. This certified RPA has provided an excellent explanation of what a RPA and a RA are and what each can offer a radiology department. She expresses her motivated interest so radiologists, fellow RPA's, student RPA's, and interested radiographers can develop an understanding of how this new group of advanced trained technologists can improve productivity and provide excellent patient care by performing procedures that consume large segments of time in a normal duty day of a radiologist.

RPA/RA's can perform fluoroscopy, angiography, and other invasive procedures. The use of a RPA/RA in radiology reduces costs, increases reimbursements, and decreases patient wait time.

In her manual, Ms. Oberoi eloquently outlines what RPA students can expect to experience from the application phase, the studying time, the traveling period, the effected home-life experiences, the certification board study segment, and the employment phase. She has prepared a wonderful manuscript in an autobiographical form that is altruistic.

Based on her trials and tribulations of being one of the first fifty RPA's certified by the Certification Board of Radiology Practitioner Assistants (CBRPA), the author provides solutions to most questions asked by any interested radiographer about a RPA/RA and for any radiologist, who asks, "What is a Radiology Practitioner Assistant or a Radiology Assistant and what can they do for me?"

This text will be a great aid that can guide a future RPA/RA student, a current RPA/RA student and the certified Radiology Practitioner Assistants and Radiology Assistants.

Charles O Williams, B.S., RPA, RT (R), (CV), (CI)

PREFACE

There I was, a 12 year veteran of radiology looking for something more than cross- training into yet another modality, when a visiting Radiology Practitioner Assistant (RPA) introduced me to Weber State University and Jane Van Valkenburg. I had so many misconceptions about the school, the program and how the RPA education could truly benefit me. I had read some articles in radiology magazines to prepare myself, but what was I to believe? Who was giving me the correct advice? My only realistic option was to contact the one and only school which was offering the RPA program at the time. Dr. Jane Van Valkenburg at Weber State University was eager to help a frightened yet resolved radiologic technologist from Austin, Texas. After years of graduating successful RPAs her advice was sound and optimistic. What a comforting person she was at a time where there was so much confusion among the "know it alls" in radiology. Jane sent me articles and necessary legislative resolves which ensured me that this was the up and coming field in radiology. This is what I was hoping for and I am so glad I followed her advice. I researched and then later prepared a RPA education proposal for my employer. I presented the information to the right people. This took strength, commitment and the resolve to not give up. After committee votes and funding clarifications, my wish was finally granted. My education was funded and I was given a chance to learn and practice my new skills. When I graduated from Weber State University in March of 2002, I was the first and only RPA in Texas. This was a little lonely, yet exciting just the same. Since then I have been informed that 23 more RPAs will be joining me in Texas from Weber's program by the year 2006. What an accomplishment!

There are many confusing issues out there concerning the RPA, including the use of the name RPA vs. RA. We don't know exactly where we are going, and if we would ever get the credit we truly deserve for bringing about a much needed change in the profession. We have to remember, that we are the best of the best in radiology and Jane Van Valkenburg at Weber State is the lady with the vision. Her vision helped the large radiology associations, such as the American Society of Radiologic Technologists and the American College of Radiology to take notice and promote the emerging profession. Whether we attend the RPA or the RA programs, we are all coming from he same basic mold and the desire to be recognized for our abilities. A study conducted by Rebecca Ludwig which was published in an 8/15/03 Auntminnie.com article confirms that many radiologic technologists already perform tasks which are considered to be outside of their scope of practice. Most technologists were doing anything from obtaining consent to even giving unofficial readings to other physicians. For many years we have been guiding radiology nurses, emergency room physicians and even some of the Radiologists, while standing in the shadows, hoping for a break. Sometimes you have to create your own "break". I believe the time is finally here for us to gather our resolve and pursue what's truly in our hearts. With this, I encourage you to be the best of whatever you have wanted to be in radiology and in life. Don't give up when things may seem hopeless, because just when you think it's over, you will discover a way to circumvent yet another obstacle.

One of the most important reasons for writing this book was to help other RTs and radiology professionals understand the RPA profession. I can tell you that I am often called upon to answer questions for radiologists, administrators and other RPA students. What better way to inform my fellow RTs about what I have learned than to put it in writing? The other reason ofcourse was to give the RPA students a guide for their new adventure. If you are reading this, I already know you are a hard worker who has ambition and the drive to embark on such an adventure. If you work hard, follow the advice you have been afforded, you can overcome the challenges and enjoy the true rewards. Remember to thank the people who helped you on your journey as I now thank my family and friends along with the instructors and doctors who have helped me through my exciting and rewarding expedition. In particular I would like to thank the Radiologists at Austin Radiological Association and the staff at Weber State University. The RPAs and the students have been instrumental in inspiring me to write this book and thus my whole hearted thanks go out to them as well. God Bless.

CONTRIBUTIONS AND ACKNOWLEDGEMENTS

1. Quotes from radiologists by Scott Burton, RPA

2. Story by Eric Burd, RPA

3. Story by James Abraham, RPA

4. Proofreading by Jane Van Valkenburg, PhD, RT (R) (N) FASRT

5. Proofreading by Charles Williams, RPA

6. School liaison for information gathering - Jerri Byers

7. Many RPAs and students contributed to state law survey

TABLE OF CONTENTS

CHAPTER 1

INTRODUCTION TO THE PROFESSION

What is a Radiology Practitioner Assistant/Radiologist Assistant?
What's in the name?

A.
What is a Radiology Practitioner Assistant/ Radiologist Assistant?

The Radiology Practitioner Assistants and the Radiologist Assistants are newly emerging allied health care professionals who are providing a recognized advanced clinical role for experienced radiologic technologists. The American College of Radiology and American Society of Radiologic Technologists, along with the National Society of Radiology Practitioner Assistants and Weber State University have worked together to facilitate the continuing growth of this profession.

Thus far, the RPAs have been performing under the supervision of the attending radiologist and working in hospitals and outpatient clinical environments. Special procedures in angiography and cardiac catheterization suites, fluoroscopy, and minor invasives such as biopsies and lumbar punctures are just some of the areas in which RPAs thrive. There is no hard fast rule as to what these radiologist extenders can or can not do. The formal guidelines from the education gurus have been as follows:

"Working under the direct supervision of a radiologist, an advanced-level radiologic technologist (RA/RPA) would take increased responsibility for patient assessment, patient education and patient management. The RA would perform appropriate fluoroscopic and other radiology procedures under direction of the supervising radiologist, and they would also make initial imaging observations that would be conveyed to the radiologist."

Further consensus reports included lumbar puncture and biopsy type invasive procedures to be included in the scope of practice. The practice of radiology changes with every ACR meeting and new practice data analysis that becomes available. Hospital credentialing can most certainly dictate the extender's role in the radiology practice in addition to the radiologists for whom they work. The RPA must carry the necessary malpractice insurance and can not practice out-side of their scope of practice. This is established by the Certification Board for Radiology Practitioner Assistants and can vary for the new graduates of the RA program. The RAs do not have the CBRPA as their board and will need to take the American Registry for Radiologic Technologist's (ARRT) certification exam and then follow the Scope of practice established by the ASRT and ACR. There is a Powerpoint presentation on the ASRT web site (www.asrt.org) which can be very helpful in introducing you to this new field in radiology. The presentation and a consensus paper were the result of a joint meeting which took place in 2002, between the ASRT and the

ACR. After getting approval from the ACR, the ASRT offered grants to schools to start developing the RA program.

These schools were offered grants by the ASRT to start their RA programs:

Loma Linda University-started 2003

Midwestern State University-started 2004

University of North Carolina at Chapel Hill

University of Medicine and Dentistry of New Jersey

These schools did not receive grant money, but have decided to consider offering the RA Program

Bloomsburg University of Pennsylvania

Massachusetts College of Pharmacy and Health Sciences

Ohio State University

Quinnipiac University

S.U.N.Y. Upstate Medical University

University of Alabama at Birmingham

Virginia Commonwealth University

I have researched the tuition rates and contact information for all of these schools. They are listed in later chapters. I did find that most of the schools that did not get the grants had not set up their programs online yet. More programs will be starting in the fall of 2005. Massachusetts College of Pharmacy and Health Sciences and Virginia Commonwealth University will also offer their RA program with a BS degree, while Bloomsburg University will offer a master's level program. There is another RPA program at South College in Knoxville, TN and it offers a master's level study as well. The Weber State RPA program is still waiting for the approval to add the master's level designation to their existing RPA program. I will be adding more information as it becomes available to me. You are also welcome to e-mail me for current information at bovna_rpa1@verizon.net

You must realize that the Weber state RPA program has had the chance to work out most of the bugs, because they have been providing this program for almost a decade! The tuition rates for the Weber State University program were the least expensive of any other school after considerable research and they offer two classes per year, instead of one, which gives more students a chance to participate in the RPA program. It is your choice on how you want to get there, as long as it is right for you.

As you can see, the profession will soon be in the main stream of radiology, at least academically speaking. Being one of the firsts in any field has its' advantages. You can make up the rules as you go along and mold your practice to what best suits your abilities and desires. As more and more schools follow in the footsteps of Weber State University, your chances of finding an affordable and convenient RPA/RA program will become more feasible. I will have to admit with all biases aside, that the Weber State RPA program is by far one of the most affordable programs that exist.

B.
What's in the name?

Many of the RPAs have wondered why the Weber State University RPA program and the RPA name did not fair well with the media or the radiology associations as it should have? Maybe it was poor marketing or the fact the educators wanted the RPAs to get into the field undetected. Sending RPAs under the radar gave the RPAs ability to grow without alarming predators in their habitat. The university did approach the ASRT when the program began in the 90s, but they were dismissed due to supposed personal differences and political pressures. Dr. Jane Van Valkenburg tried to get them involved numerous times, but the political environment was just not quite right for the largest supporting Radiologic Technologist society (ASRT) to pursue the RPA issue. After all it was not in the mainstream of thought. Jane continued to train the RPAs and kept hoping that one day the American College of Radiology and ASRT would see the potential. Fear as well as the loss of control spawned by the increasing number of RPAs in practice gave rise to the first conference held in 2002, to discuss the issue and to approve what the ACR thought was a good name and guidelines for practice. This was over five years after the first RPAs had graduated; The National Society of Radiology Practitioner Assistants was already increasing in membership and holding national conferences to educate their own without any help from their radiology counterparts.

I was just standing in the sidelines observing as my future was being decided by people who had no idea of how the RPA practice actually worked. I was a RPA student at the time and had to battle my own battles due to this joint meeting. Before the consensus paper was made public, I was in a hospital network being trained and was performing most tasks generally performed by the radiologists. Some of the radiologists preferred that I perform these tasks, not only to gain experience, but because I was better at performing them than they were. Not meaning to sound conceited, but a radiologic technologist with over 12 years of experience has some insight into what a procedure entails and can do a great job performing it. I can certainly see that fear may have played a big role in the ACR's disapproval of the RPA name, after all our counterparts in the United Kingdom have made a great practice for themselves. The radiologic technologists of advanced practice in England can not only perform procedures, but they can dictate and bill for services much like our nurse practitioners and physician assistants. The radiologist association assumed that the otherwise loyal radiologic technologists turned RPAs who had worked along side the radiologists all of these years, would now go out on their own and compete with the radiologists for jobs and medical market share. Further, it was thought that the RPAs would go to the competing fields such as vascular surgery and cardiology.

Radiologists had already been loosing turf battles to the vascular surgeons and cardiologists and anyone else who wanted to practice radiology. It was so easy to put a MRI and CT scanner along with an ultrasound unit in their offices and offer these services to their own patients. Not to mention the interventional procedures being performed in the hospitals by these specialists. The radiologists failed to see that one of the reasons they were loosing these turf battles was, because there was a decrease in the radiologist pool as many of the publications have pointed out. Also, the radiology reports were not getting out on time and there were not enough radiologists for consultation. This has been the subject of many news articles and conferences for the radiologists and the specialists such as cardiologists and vascular surgeons. I feel that the specialized physicians had no choice, but to take the matter into their own hands. Their own professional societies started putting out papers and encouraged them to learn about radiology to help their patient flow. The radiologists can't totally blame these specialists when the radiologists themselves were the catalysts for such a reaction

Further, as the number of exams increased, the daily pathology become more complex and the technology grew at an enormous rate, the radiologists found themselves working harder than ever. In fact as a radiologist from a major children's hospital talks about this issue of increased workload and decrease in radiologists in the article "Hunting for recruits, pediatric radiologists take aim at "misconceptions" published on the Auntminnie web site on 6/2/03. To summarize, it was stated that imaging has grown 10 times what was predicted and it is mainly due to trying to reduce costs of hospital stay. Since doctors want to release the patients as soon as they are better, hence they are prescribing more imaging studies to help them make a clearer decision. Further, over the years the primary care physicians have become the "gatekeepers of what is ordered and this will ensure that more tests will be ordered." Another article titled "Imaging by non-radiologists drives up healthcare costs" by Leslie Farnsworth dated 11/25/02 from the Auntminnie website suggests that imaging by non radiologists is growing by leaps and bounds. Furthermore it is driving up healthcare costs, because some of this imaging is either unnecessary and or only driven by financial gain. A study performed by Dr. David C Levin, former chairperson of radiology at Thomas Jefferson University Hospital in Philadelphia found that the work billed by radiologists from 1993 to 1999 had increased only 7 percent for Medicare patients where non-radiologists' billing was over 32 percent!

Most radiologists still work about 10-12 hour days and then pull call and have to rotate through the weekends. The salaries of the radiologist are growing just as any other radiology professional, since there is more demand than the supply. The larger groups are able to cover the costs of these huge salaries, but some of the other practices are not fairing so well. Some practices have told me that it's not that they are interviewing the employee candidates, but being interviewed themselves. And if the radiology can't meet a candidate's demands, they just go to someone who will. Most radiology groups are in fact trying to do more with fewer radiologists, just for this very reason. Another issue is timely manner in which the reports are going out to the referring physicians and the ability to market effectively. The report turn-around times are now being made to be monitored by experts and marketing is playing a big role in trying to keep the remaining imaging business. Unfortunately, this has also lead to a marked increase in costs to run a radiology practice and decreases the ability for the less fortunate group's survival. With the advent of the Picture Archiving and communications System (PACS), radiologists are able to cover more facilities and get the reports out faster to the specialists.

Even though the radiologists may be keeping up with the times with respect to technological and administrative aspects, they lack in the workforce arena. While they are working through their problems, the radiologists never really stopped to look at how the other medical practices have evolved to overcome the physician shortages and reduce costs. If the Radiologists don't start looking at the RPA as a solution more of the same old problems will persist. A Diagnostic Imaging article sums this up nicely in the April 2004 issue, which states that, "Staffing shortages imply a lack of balance between the available workforce and the work that is needed to deliver a service. Possible solutions involve increasing the workforce or decreasing the workload. If neither is done, staff members will be unhappy, recruitment problems will arise, and fewer people will be available to do the work. As a result, radiology will not be able to deliver a quality service, and other specialties will invade our turf."

As some of the other educators have been pointing out that radiology is just not very attractive to new recruits in medicine. The Radiologists are seen as being run down and overworked especially in an academic setting where it leaves the faculty radiologists very little or no real time to teach the residents. As an academic radiologist points out in a recent article, "Hunting for recruits, pediatric radiologists take aim at misconceptions" dated 6/26/03, "attracting more Radiologists means creating a positive environment, one in which radiologists have time to teach the residents properly. Research time must be protected and encouraged, vacation time increased, call frequency reduced. Hiring more staff such as ACR-trained Radiologist Assistants will reduce interruptions, ease the administrative burden, and make radiologists more productive." The complete article can be seen on www. Auntminnie.com

There are physician's assistants and nurse practitioners in virtually every medical specialty. Because there were no physician extenders in radiology, the PAs and the NPs found their way easily into the radiology arena. If I would have been in their place, I may have done the same thing. Why not? I don't believe there should be any hard feelings toward these professionals, just because of their role. We didn't exist as radiology extenders just yet, so they stepped in. Furthermore the radiologists found themselves training these paraprofessionals in the art of radiology with the help of the radiologic technologists. Like a new language, they would have to either start from scratch or have them perform only limited tasks which can be easily done by a radiology nurse and a special procedures technologist. I don't think that most radiologists really figured out how to utilize these persons. They trained them and let them perform tasks which would help ease the radiologist burden.

I can't really expect an overworked radiologist to put together a training program along with trying to keep his/her head just above water. Moreover as the shortage of radiologists reached critical mass, the radiologists had no time to think outside the box. They grabbed who ever was available and willing to be trained. Having realized that, I also don't understand why so many radiologists didn't see the potential in the special procedures technologists who assisted them day in and day out. They should have seen that these assistants who had been supplementing them everyday would have a niche for this. I do believe that a few radiologists did see their potential, but used it to have them train the nurse practitioners and physician's assistants who where their recent hire. This may have been due to the lack of recognition of the RPAs and the ability to bill for service by other mid-level providers. Some of the RPAs have confessed to me that they have had to train PAs and NPs in the angiography suite to perform tasks which were actually considered as the natural progression of a radiologic technologist. Most of my peers have stated that they had already been performing such tasks and now there was an outsider here to take their place. It's only natural to bear resentment toward a situation such as this. Most RTs just kept their mouth shut and quietly disapproved of the whole situation.

Paying another salary to train someone else to perform tasks which could easily and more safely be performed by the radiologist physician extender just seemed wasteful to most special procedures technologists I have spoken with. Further, as I found out at a recent conference, these newly trained PAs and NPs can and have taken these new skills and marketed them to the highest bidder. It is true that the radiologists have to train the radiology technologist to perform more complicated tasks, but at least we speak the same language. As one of my radiologists tells everyone, "she won't leave us like residents after she is trained. We get to keep her for a while." A radiology trained PA or a NP is very valuable to another specialist trying to embrace the radiology practice. The laws for billing for radiology procedures are already in place and there is nothing stopping them from leaving the radiologist and going elsewhere. It's true that there are movements to reverse some of these, but either way, since they have been around longer and have more members for influence, it's just a matter of time. Contracts between radiologists and these professionals have curtailed some of the moves to other specialties, but a contract can't hold someone forever. Therefore, by keeping the name to reflect that the radiology physician extender would practice only under a radiologist (RA) the ACR hopes to prevent the RAs from working with other specialties with or without a binding contract.

RPAs are working all across the United States and finding job prospects to be very good. From the east cost to the west coast, the RPAs are being snatched up by busy radiology practices.

Many work in hospitals in the interventional suites others in outpatient clinics and small community hospitals. They do work along side the radiologists and have become good friends with their employers. Some have become such good friends that they come to the NSRPA conferences and hold workshops together. The radiologists who employ the RPAs can definitely see the value and this has led to a major increase in the salary range for the RPA since the first graduates arrived at the scene. The salary average in the mid 1990s was about $65K, which has now risen to $90K, with some RPAs making in excess of $125K and being offered partnerships. Recently, I have been notified that the RA programs are looking for more RPAs to teach their students and be directors of their RA programs. Kiser Permanente and other healthcare businesses are starting to advertise for the RPA positions. There are efforts to get another major hospital system to make the RPA/RA a part of their medical team across the United States. We've come a long way and it's only going to get better.

There are still many more hurdles coming our way. Will the RPA and RA be merged under one umbrella? Will the RPA be a master's level and the RA a BS degree? Will the RPAs be able to do more than the RA? Will there be another society for the RAs? Will we have our own Medicare PIN numbers for billing? Radiologists and hospital administrators seem to feel better if we can bill on our own. All of these concepts are being entertained. As with any other new and progressive entity, we have the chance to mold it into what will benefit us in the future. By being involved you can assure that you will have a say in this, otherwise you will have to accept what becomes of your profession. We can't point fingers at the ASRT or the ACR for forming policy when we don't stand up for our selves. Maybe they have not seen the solution that we see, or they see problems that we can not. We do have to work together as a team. There will be many battles to fight with the Medicare billing issues and other supporting issues. We have to consider the ASRT and the ACR as our partners.

What's in the name? Well, not too much. One just came before the other. The RPAs were visionaries who took a chance on a potential they saw and the RAs played it safe and waited for the concept to be main stream before committing to it. There is nothing wrong with either choice. Some of us are gamblers and some like to play it safe. The RPAs do deserve the credit and I think most of the RA programs totally agree. Whatever has been done in the past remains in the past, but we can learn from it and move ahead. RPA and RAs communicate on a regular basis, and the RAs have been seen attending the RPA society meeting last year in 2004. I hope they will make a point to attend many more meetings in the future. The RPAs are helping some of the RA programs with education. Some RPAs are working as consultants for these programs and some are being asked to teach classes and help with clinicals. We have been working together and we will keep working together to promote the radiologist extenders as opposed to having other extenders move into a feuding family. Now that we can agree that we are essentially the same, let's move forward.

NOTES (WHAT IS THE RPA/RA ABOUT)

CHAPTER 2
THE CHOICES

How to evaluate a RPA/RA program

Before you start, what to consider (Jobs, Money, Family, Moving)

Are you ready to move forward for the right reasons?

A.

How to evaluate a **RPA/RA** program

Now that you know that the Radiologist Extender is a feasible solution in the eyes of many radiologists, which program will you attend? There are a number of things you should look for in a good RA/RPA program. As with any new concept, there is a bit of experimentation until consistency is achieved. With all of these new RA programs starting out, why then do students flock to the Weber State RPA program? There is a little uncertainty of a RA/RPA merge or even the level of acceptance which may be gained from becoming a RPA rather than a RA. The answer is simple. Weber State has offered the Program for about a Decade and has had continued success with their RPAs. Not to say that the RA programs will not have similar success with the RAs, but there is a standard you should look for.

1. Geographic location-You have to be able to attend

2. Reputation of the school and implementation of the RPA/RA program

3. Courses being offered

    a. Pathophysiology, pharmacology, radiobiology, federal regulations, and fluoroscopy

    b. Cross Sectional Anatomy and computerized imaging

    c. Radiology procedures including invasive studies, clinical decision making/ pathways and problem patient management

    d. Ethics and medico legal courses, psycho-social medicine, patient education, and patient assessment

    e. Evaluation of all human body systems, clinical preceptorship and competency assessment

    f. Research requirement and teaching current trends

4. Cost-If you have to pay for it yourself

    a. scholarship programs and financial aid

5. A good student network for support

6. Graduation requirements

    a. BS degree preferred if you do not already have one

No matter which school you choose, if you do the research you can't be misled. The ASRT website has updates on their educational proposals for the RA programs and you can go to the CBRPA we site for RPA curriculum. You will find that being a RPA or RA you will be doing lots and lots of research. We are heading into a new territory and we have to make the pathway and stick to it.

B.

BEFORE YOU START, WHAT TO CONSIDER
(JOBS, MONEY, FAMILY, MOVING)

After being in radiology for many years, you may have wondered about a different life. One that is even more fulfilling than the one you have become accustomed to. How do you make this change and where do you start? You might have many reservations about a profession that is riddled with conflictions and can't even agree on its' professional title. Hopefully, I can put your mind at ease and help you discover if this journey is right for you.

Before we talk about the challenges, let's discuss your needs. Everyone has their own set of values and needs that are specific to their environment and region of the country. I would recommend that you form a list of the things you would like to keep the same and the ones you want to change (sort of a self-evaluation). This does not only include professional wishes, but personal ones as well. Only you can establish what these requirements are, and how important each one is to your life. Some of these things might be; work environment, family, geographical location, money, direction of career. Once you have your list then start reading the rest of this book to see if this is what you really want. We did have some people in my class who did not want to be a part of this and decided to leave after the first class. Sometimes it was the salary range, other times it was the time requirement for studying and the compulsory dedication. Whatever their reasons were, they wasted not only their time, but the time of the school and the chance for another student to be in the class. Hopefully you can understand why you must try your best to avoid a similar scenario. Try talking with your family members, especially your husband or wife, before you actually apply to the school. You may even want someone else to read this book and application materials to gain a dual perspective. You, your self, may even have a clouded judgment, because you may really want to attend the program. Whatever you decide to do, I hope this book will serve as a good reference and give you the opportunity to make the correct decision.

Now that you can approach this with some objectivity, we can consider some of the basic necessities. There are some requirements set by the Radiology Practitioner Assistant/Radiologist's Assistant programs which ensure that the student base will have adequate radiology experience before matriculation. The program at Weber State University (WSU) requires that you must have at least five years of radiology experience as a radiologic technologist, before matriculation. This means that you can apply to the program before completing five years, as long as you will have five years under your belt when you start the program in the fall. The deadline is usually in

December of the year prior to matriculation, but may vary depending on the school you choose. You will also need a computer with high speed internet access, since most of your tests will be on-line. Why the high speed connection? Well, when you are looking at images and trying to answer questions within the time allotted, you want every advantage possible. Many students in the past have tried to take their tests with a dial-up modem, but finally had to switch to high speed access.

Requirements in general:

1. Two-five years as a full-time radiologic technologist

2. ARRT Certification, state license if needed

3. BCLS and ACLS

4. Completed application to school and program by due date

5. High speed Internet access

6. Time and place to do clinicals (some schools provide preceptors)

When I have discussed this opportunity with fellow radiology technologists, the first thing they ask me is, "How much will I get paid?" and next, "How much will it cost?" With so many opportunities for overtime these days, I can certainly understand monetary reluctances. I have worked two and three jobs and counted on overtime wages to pay the bills myself. If money is the only thing that is driving you toward the RPA/RA, then this may not be the right adventure for you. Most people don't realize that the RPA is a salaried position and even though it may be highly lucrative for some, it may not be for you. I won't even talk about the marketing issues which may be involved. The salary ranges vary depending on your region and the opportunity to make $85K or above in 2004 is very promising. You can also log on to www.CBRPA.org and see the current salary ranges for your region of the country. The general rule of thumb is double what you're making now. Like with anything else, after you have built a good foundation, then you can enjoy the rewards. You will have to do some hard work by propositioning radiologists and hospitals to let you practice as a student and later as a full fledged RPA. The first two years can be tasking, but very feasible if you are patient.

In keeping with the money theme, the cost of the program varies due to travel costs. In my opinion the cost of the WSU RPA program is very reasonable for most students. Depending on your geographic location, you have to factor in flights, hotel stay and meals. Citing the Weber State example, I can tell you about my experiences. I would usually get to Salt Lake City on Wednesday night and get a rental car for the three days I was there. Some students, who arrived together on the same day and around the same time, could share rental cars. You will definitely need a car rental, because the school is about an hour drive from the Salt Lake City airport. You will travel to school 3 times in the first semester, two times for three more semesters and the summer semester trip is optional, but recommended. This puts your flight count at 9-10. Hotel can cost you anywhere from $50-$80 per night for three nights at a time. Some students also shared rooms and this can also cut your costs significantly. Meals always depend on a person's eating habits, so you will have to figure this out for your self. I tried to have some non perishables with me so that I could eat these for short lunches. You can always choose to go out for lunch, but sometimes there wasn't enough time, before the next class. There are many nice restaurants, but then there are fast food places as well. For dinner, I would usually go out with other RPA students. There is also, a small cost for parking at the university, so you can figure about $5-6 for that. The fall and spring trips can be freezing sometimes, so check the weather before you go. You may want to invest in some winter clothing, if you do not have some.

All in all, I had asked my employer for a $15,000 budget, which was sufficient to cover my entire education expense. The tuition has gone up $200 per semester at Weber State since I attended, but still reasonable. If you want my advice, the trade off is well worth it. Most of the time, you can contact your group of radiologists or a competitive radiology group and ask them to sponsor your education. I know of many RPAs who did exactly that. You may want to reference the pertinent sections of this book before finding sponsorship and funding.

Here's the breakdown of costs:

1. Tuition $8500 (Current)

2. Books and modules $1500

3. Travel $4500

4. Computer expenses $500

This total comes to $16,000 (Weber example)

Many of us who are old veterans of radiology have a family to take care of, and this is where one may have to sacrifice. For the next five semesters you will be immersed in radiology and your family will either support it or hate it. This is something I truly believe one should discuss, before even contacting the school. I was able to juggle home and the rigorous requirements of being an RPA student because of the lack of children in my life. However, there have been many women in the program who did have demanding family responsibilities to focus on. They found it difficult, but doable, especially when their husbands stepped up and supported them through it. For the men in the program, it may be a little easier than ladies. From the family aspect everyone's needs vary and you are the only one who can decide if you and your family can live through this career evolution. Have your significant other read at least this chapter of the book, if not all of it, so that they may understand the process and help you make the decision. Who knows? They may even support you and appreciate you for taking on such a task to make a better future for them and yourself.

I have been asked, "Does the student need to move to Utah to study?" There is no need to move closer to the school. This not only makes it easier for you with family matters, but helps you with establishing a preceptorship. Staying close to a community in which you have already built good relationships, has its' rewards. Maybe the hospital radiology group wants to train you and help you with the tuition? If you move away from a community to save on travel costs, you are not looking at this with a keen eye. Moves can be very expensive and living with relatives can leave you very stressed. You don't want to uproot your family on top of other program stresses. Stay where you are, do this with distance learning and get your radiologists to pay for it. This is my message.

C.

ARE YOU READY TO MOVE FORWARD FOR THE RIGHT REASONS?

Before you decide you want to move on with your career, analyze your situation and remember what you discovered in your self-evaluation. Many radiologic technologists are merely burnt out and are looking for a change. Sometime the RPA can be enough of a change, but sometimes it can be a waste of time to make you more miserable. Some people have expressed to me the inability to tolerate any more call hours. It is possible that you may one day cover call for a radiology group, but this is not the norm. I do think that the increasing demand and the short supply of RPA/RAs enables us to dictate our working conditions and the hours worked in a day. You will have to talk this over with your radiology group, but don't forget to consider the negotiation section in this book, before you do decide to approach the radiologists. Below are some symptoms of burnout.

If you are truly burned out, find out what the source of this is. If it is the radiology field, you may not want to spend time and energy to attend RPA/RA program. There will be a time in the beginning of your clinicals where you will wonder where you fit in and if you are not able to tackle this with emotional stability, it will be a disaster. I have met some technologists who just wanted to do something else. When I have questioned them, they have expressed the desire to take a desk job or get out of the health field all together. They did not want to however, waste their medical training. The RPA does give you other areas to expand into, but you may wind up working in a similar environment as the one you may have dreaded. Take some time and consider the symptoms carefully and be sure you are doing this for the right reasons.

1. Chronic fatigue - exhaustion, tiredness, a sense of being physically run down

2. Anger at people making demands

3. Self-criticism for putting up with the demands

4. Cynicism, negativity, and irritability

5. A sense of being overwhelmed

6. Exploding easily at seemingly unimportant things

7. Recurrent headaches and gastrointestinal disturbances

8. Weight loss or gain

9. Sleeplessness and depression

10. Shortness of breath

11. Suspiciousness

12. Feelings of vulnerability

13. Increased degree of risk taking

What I would do is to make a list of everything that bothers you about your job situation in the status quo/at present. Compare them to the list above which was compiled after reading the article "Tell tail signs of Burnout" by: Dore De Gray, with specific examples. If you can figure out what bothers you and brings out a symptom from the above list, then you can be ready to evaluate it and see if being a RPA/RA will alleviate this symptom, or make it worse. I too have had some issues with burnout and wanted to share this with you.

I have found some coping skills to work well for me and I will offer these to you now. The first thing to do, as I mentioned above is, find the source of the stress. Next, try developing some ways to relieve stress. You can find this on www.helpguide.com. Just by organizing your life, taking breaks and nurturing yourself, you can make a big difference. You may have too many things going on which can be organized or shared with a family member. If this is at work, try designating some tasks to others who are capable. I know this takes trust, but in the long run you will win out like I have. This will also enable you to take vacations with your family and a chance to recharge. Don't be so hard on your self. I had to learn this painfully and over time. Also, by keeping a diary, you can relieve some stress and monitor your progress. Most people think diaries are for little girls and young children, but they are so much more powerful than you can imagine. How can you fix something when you can't even find the cause? Keeping a journal whether it's actually hand written or on a computer, can help you organize your thoughts, let alone have you discover what they are. It just made sense to me and I did it. Maybe it will help you too. Some issues are so insidious and hidden that we can't put a finger on them. And by the time they affect us to the point it's intolerable, we may need some professional help. I can tell you that writing this book has been very therapeutic and inspirational for me. I would also suggest that if you have some issues that come up and bother you, please try discussing this with your family doctor. So many of us try to deal with private issues our selves, but I found my doctor to a tremendous help. I only wished that I had resources to diagnose this earlier in my RPA adventure and I hope this helps you in that regard. Once you know how the RPA position will affect you, you can move forward and decide when to proceed.

NOTES (CHOICES AVAILABLE)

CHAPTER 3
THE NECESSITIES

How to apply to the program
Here are helpful contacts for your journey through the profession
Overcoming your fears-Laws and billing practices
Setting up a preceptorship and keeping it

A.

How to apply to the program

No matter which radiology practitioner assistant or radiologist's assistant program you choose, you will have to show the desire and the commitment to be considered a good applicant. With the rising demand for the RPA/RA programs and the low number of programs that exist, you will need to stand out from the rest of the students. I can only talk about the Weber State RPA program and my knowledge of the Midwestern State University RA programs.

Once you have made the decision to attend a specific program, you must make contact with the school whether it is via e-mail or by phone. If you decide on Weber State University, you should send an e-mail to Jerri Byers. Her address is listed on the helpful contacts chapter. I have also given you information on how to apply to the RA program at Midwestern state university on the contacts page. Once Jerri receives your request, she or one of her staff members will send out a packet to your home via US mail. When you first receive your packet of information along with the application, make sure you inventory the items. Make sure you have the application to apply to the university itself and the RPA program. There will be some helpful information about the program and the timeline for the selection process included with the packet. Read through everything and contact Jerri if you have any questions. You can also go on to the university web site and gather more information about the program. Remember you can always get some of your questions answered via the CBRPA web site.

Make sure you get all of your paperwork in order. Obtain your transcripts and get them to the University. Use the address which is provided. You don't want to send them to the wrong department. They generally go to the Radiologic Sciences department with attention to the RPA program. Your prior radiologic technology school or other higher education institution will have their own procedures to follow. You will have to fill out a transcript release form and there is usually a charge for the actual official transcript to be sent to your new school. You may want to get an unofficial transcript for your records as well. I have had to refer to my old transcripts at least a dozen times in the past fifteen years. They come in handy when you need them. Check on-line at www.weber.edu to see if you meet any of the core competency requirements already. General Education Core competencies are the courses you will need to qualify for graduation with a certain degree. Whether you are going for your BS degree or master's, it is a good idea to see what all of the requirements exists for graduation. This way you can plan your didactic study timeline. One thing I would recommend is that you try to get some of the classes you will need at the community college in your home town. You will be able to take non radiology classes at your own pace at Weber state, but it will be at a cost of out of state tuition. So, I actually took my Art and computer classes needed to graduate, in Austin. You can do this as well and save a little money and time. You should also, contact the distant learning office to make sure you are following all of their rules. You can accomplish this by calling Weber State University and asking the operator to connect you to the distance learning office. It is that easy. Talk with the secretaries at the Radiologic Sciences office and confirm you have everything they have sent to you.

Make certain you have at least three references and that they are all from the radiologists for whom you have worked. Even though the application may ask for one supervisor recommendation, go ahead and add this as an extra. The committee wants to know if you have support from the radiologists. The reference forms are provided to you in the packet and you should have them sent to the school by January 15th following the December 1st deadline. If you follow this book, it should take you just a Saturday afternoon to fill out the application and plan for transcripts and reference letters.

Continuing with the application, there is a portion on the in which you are asked to list all of your employment for the past years. You must make a list of all jobs and any gaps in employment. Make a list of all schools and programs you have attended. If there are gaps in the timeline show why there are gaps and what you did during that time. You will get an opportunity to write an autobiography and these lists will help you when you come to this part of the application. Remember the selection committee is looking for someone who stands out from the rest, but they are also looking for someone who has not only overcome adversity, but someone who is stable and consistent academically. The first semester can be pretty rough, so show how well you can write along with the experienced thought process which you possess. The selection committee does not know you as a person and it is your job to show them via the essay what a great person you are and what immense contributions you may make to the profession. Most people hate writing essays, but think about it. After writing all of those essays in school for just a grade, now writing one that can actually make a real difference in your life. Have someone proof read it even if you don't want them to see it. It is better that they help you fix a mistake, than to have the selection committee do it.

If you have any questions or you want some reassurance, contact a fellow RPA. If you can not find one, contact me. One thing you will find in the RPA community is that everyone wants you to do well and they <u>will</u> help you. We are all very busy with our jobs and families, but if you are trying hard to succeed, we will see it and help you along.

Here is a quick guide to filling out the application and the time required:

Weber State Application: Short form (30mins, longer if you don't have prior high school and university information)

RPA Application: Some repetition of the Weber State University application and work experience (30-45mins)

RPA application communication portion: Listed below are the questions asked on the typical application.

1. Reason(s) for desiring to enter the program

2. List your strengths and weaknesses

3. What you most enjoy doing in your leisure time

4. One thing you have accomplished that has given you great satisfaction

5. Any other information about yourself which you feel is pertinent to the application

These questions may not be the same for you, but my experience has been that most programs have similar requests. Most people also consider me to be a professional student.

Applying to any of the RA programs will depend on your preference and location of residence. The Midwestern State University in Texas is great for the Texas residents. The program costs approximately $3000 in tuition and book expenses per semester. This is for in-state tuition only and it doubles to $6000 for out of state students. These figures were taken from their web site on Sep 23 2004. Loma Linda University in California charges $20K- $24K for their RA programs as listed on their web site. Completion time is 21 months or 7 quarters and you can choose from two options. You can get a certificate, if you already possess a bachelor's or you can get a bachelor's when you graduate. The program tuition thus far has been in the $15K-20K range for in state students. Some of the out of state tuitions were as high as $16K per semester and this did not include books. Weber State's program asked for a special authorization to allow the RPA students to have the in-state status. This has kept the tuition very low at about $1700 per semester. You just can't beat this!

When you have decided where you want to attend, look at the schools web site and weigh your options carefully. Making a few long distance phone calls to the program directors, are highly recommended. Moreover, you may want to contact some of the RPAs or the RAs who are practicing and get the skinny on the schools. I have discovered that Massachusetts College of Pharmacy and Health Sciences and Bloomsburg University will be offering their programs in 2005. Bloomberg offers a masters level RA program, but they require that at least two semesters be on campus. I have received confirmation that Virginia Commonwealth University will also offer their program in 2005. They were very quick to send me a complete packet for entrance into the program.

Weber State University has been trying to upgrade their RPA program to a master's level, but it seems this will not happen until 2005 or 2006. There is a master's level RPA program which will be offered by South College in Knoxville, TN. Weber State has been elicited to help with this also. I discovered the education approval and funding document for this program, via the web on Sep 23 2004. The program name is RPA and a Master of Science will be awarded to the graduates. The program length is 100 quarter hours or 88 weeks. This was approved by the Tennessee higher education commission on July 15 2004.

As new programs are being offered, do your homework and pick the one that is best for you. After checking the curriculum for the four programs that received the ASRT grants, I have not seen much uniformity. They are using different admission criteria, different books and can't agree on which courses to teach. They will learn by trial and error and hopefully in a few years, some uniformity will be evident. Choose wisely and read the rest of the book.

B.

HERE ARE HELPFUL CONTACTS FOR YOUR JOURNEY THROUGH THE PROFESSION

The first contact is the official website for the RPAs which is

www.CBRPA.org

This site will give you information on what you can do as a RPA, what laws are there to help you, the salary ranges for RPAs and any new information which is being circulated which involves this profession.

Next, is the site for the school which will give you the RPA curriculum, so that you can decide what you have and what you need as far as the educational and degree requirements?

http://weber.edu/x13866.xml

You may also contact Jerry Byers at the radiologic sciences program she will send you the necessary information to apply for the program. Make sure you follow all of the instructions and contact Jerry or her co-workers, if you have any questions. Her e-mail address is:

JLBYERS@WEBER.EDU

The phone number to the school is:

1-801-626-6057

Toll Free 1-800-848-7770, then pick option 2 and the extension 6057.

Address is:

Weber State University

3925 University Circle

Ogden, UT 84408-3925

Here is some contact information for a school in Texas which is currently offering a Radiologist Assistant program. I was able to log on to www.mwsu.edu and then I click on the academics tab, then I picked extended education. I could then choose distance learning. Once I had that, I went to the links area on the top left hand side of the page and chose "Web Courses / Programs" This will get you to the programs and you must pick the "Bachelor of Radiologic Science" program to look at the RA program material. You can print the application and get started. The school site is a bit slow, so give your self plenty of time for research. I did find out that their first meeting for orientation is from Sunday to Wednesday at the end of September. You can access most of pertinent RA information on-line. They seem to have a very similar program to Weber State.

If you can get the site below to work, use this first.

http://hs2.mwsu.edu/radsci

Radiologic Sciences Department Chair

Midwestern State University

3410 Taft Blvd

Wichita Falls, Texas 76308

1-866-575-4305

Loma Linda University

www.llu.edu

University of medicine and dentistry at New Jersey

www.umdnj.edu

University of North Carolina at Chapel Hill

www.med.unc.edu

Below are some more RA and RPA program contact information which was obtained via school websites

Massachusetts College of Pharmacy and Health Sciences

Radiography Program Director

179 Longwood Avenue

Boston, MA 02115-5896

Phone: (617) 732-2820

Bloomsburg University

Professor, Biology & Allied Health

Allied Health Coordinator

104 Hartline Science Center

400 East 2nd Street

Bloomsburg, PA 17815

Phone: 570-389-4319

There is also a national society for radiology practitioner assistants, which has a very useful web site through which you can get answers to frequently asked questions and find helpful links to obtain further information. You can also register for their national conference which has been held in Las Vegas for the last 5-6 years.

The NSRPA's site is: www.radiologypa.org

There are other websites listed below which warrant some investigation on your part, but are well worth the effort and time spent. I have found them to be very helpful, when trying to find conferences, speakers, administrator's point of view and ways to expand my role as a RPA.

www.ASRT.org American Society for Radiologic Technologists

www.AHRAcom American Healthcare Radiology Administrators

www.ARRS.org American Roentgen Ray Society

www.ACR.org American college of Radiology

www.ARRT.org American Registry for Radiologic Technologists

www.RSNA.ORG Radiologic Society of North America

www.JRADIOLOOGY.com Journal of Radiology

www.Auntminnie.com The great radiology web site

C.

Overcoming your fears
Laws and billing practices

When I was first considering the RPA School, I wanted something in writing which blessed the RPA and allowed me to practice in Texas. I was not able to get such assurances. Great strides have been made in the last few years and I am very confident that the RPA profession will indeed thrive. As you may have read in the radiology journals, the American Society for Radiologic Technologists (ASRT), the American College of Radiology (ACR) and the National Society for Radiology Practitioner Assistants (NSRPA) along with other involved parties has fully supported the concept of radiologist extenders. You can access the current information on this by going to the ASRT website at www.asrt.org and the ARRT website at www.arrt.org. There is one agreement which is to our benefit, which is that the radiology extenders will not need a separate licensure as long as there are not state laws preventing delegated duties. There is also a resolve by these organizations to help change the state laws to help the extenders to practice more easily. Of course, there is the conflict with the name being used for the radiologist extenders and this will be resolved in the near future. The American Registry of Radiologic Technologists (ARRT) is sending out surveys to help draft a reasonable first draft of the roles ad responsibilities of the RA. If the RPA and RA are held to the same roles, this may limit our roles as RPAs. I have a feeling that the RAs will want to do more than the scope will initially allow and this will lead to widening of that vary scope drafted by the ARRT. It is still progress from just a year ago!

My personal experience has taught me that you should just do what you were trained to do and let the politics play themselves out. The ACR insisted that we use the title Radiologist's Assistant (RA) instead of RPA. In my opinion, there is more than one reason for this. Not only does the RA suggest that we can only work under the radiologist's supervision and no other, but by using a different label the ACR can mold the profession to their liking. I don't mind the name change, but I do mind the ACR and the ASRT using the platform founded by the Weber State University RPA program and calling it their own. I have made contact with the ASRT about this issue and although they are very kind in acknowledging us in their communiqué, they continue to promote the RA and place the RPA in a derogatory category. At times they may say a few nice things about the RPAs especially at our national meetings, but to the masses they credit themselves for coming up with the concept they so vehemently opposed in the years leading up to the extenders' recognition in the radiology community. The Weber State Program received no support from the only radiology organization which could have made a huge difference in helping the profession thrive, yet now that same society uses the same RPA curriculum and the RPAs in practice to help their project grow. It is true that WSU revived the 70s radiology PA program which did not fair well in it's time, but workforce shortages have made it imperative to pursue this option again. This time it was going to take off.

I am not angry at the concept of the RA or the persons who will be practicing as such, but I am concerned about appearances. I was happy to read that the new RAs are being interviewed for national coverage and they are proclaiming themselves as the first of such radiology extenders and best of what radiology has to offer. However, no mention is given to the struggling RPAs who took a chance on the natural evolution of the profession nine years ago and made this concept so accepted. They are the true pioneers who did not have the financial backing from their employers, no idea if they were going to get a job after they graduated and did not know that their initiative was going to be taken away from the people who started it all. I implore the new widely accepted RAs to step up and join us and stand up for what is right. Promoting a change takes courage and perseverance. Even as a student, you must make it a priority to join your true national organization, the NSRPA. Through this you can get the correct information and be able to network with your fellow RPAs and RAs. You are lucky to have a support system which did not exist until the RPAs bounded together six years ago, started the society, promoted the RPA concept and gained the necessary support for the RA to exist today. This is something to consider isn't it?

On the matter of having to obtain separate licensure, the general consensus is that we should be treated like the nurse practitioner model. After a nurse has obtained a license in a particular state and then they decide to obtain the practitioner degree, they do not obtain another license. The nurse practitioners get a special designation by the nursing board, but no new license. This is the case in Texas as I am familiar with the state and this can be confirmed from their web site. You may have to check with your state to discover how things work there. The principle is that just as the nurse practitioner credential is the extension of the nursing license, the RPA credential is the extension of the RT license.

I will have to say that the employing radiologists and the RPAs have been instrumental in breaking barriers and demanding to be recognized in many states. With the ASRT having the resolve to do the same, it is just a matter of time before we get the recognition that we desire. I recently surveyed many of the RPAs and RPA students in various sates and found some disturbing results. The most important discovery I made was that there were obvious discrepancies in how the RPAs in the same state are being treated. Mainly this was due to the lack of information available to the RPA and or the radiology group. There is a definite communication gap which has made it difficult to let the other RPAs know that they are able to practice and perform the same duties as others in the state. I have RPAs telling me that they are unable to practice and there is no state license and then a RPA from the same state lets me know that they indeed do have a license and that they were the first RPA in that same state to get a license. How bizarre?!

I know that many states are either passing new Laws specifically for the RPA/RA practice or are adding supplements to incorporate the radiologist extenders into the existing RT certification Laws. States such as Montana, Tennessee, Arkansas, and Washington are just a few who have made strides in the field. There is a misconception about New York, because I have heard at many conferences how RPAs are finding it difficult to practice. When I lived in New York several years ago, I was made aware of a "Specialist Assistant" license that was available to anyone who wanted to apply, but no one had just yet. They developed this licensure application when the first radiology assistants of the 1970's were graduating. There really shouldn't be any reason why one can not practice in New York. Recently, I have confirmation that there in fact is at least one RPA who is practicing with such license.

There exist many states which do not have even a RT license and expect the radiology community to police the ARRT registered technologists and their quality of work. Some states have actually been very RPA friendly and the RPAs are having a chance to practice as the mid-level radiology providers they were trained for. States like Colorado, Pennsylvania, North Carolina, and California have embraced RPAs and radiology practices are stocking up on them, just incase other states get wise and take them back home. We still have a long way to go, but if I look at the progress from just two years ago, when I graduated, it is immense! There is a breakdown of my state law research at the end of this section which may help you keep track of your state. If I don't have your state, please accept my apologies, for I am under time constraints.

Just as I may have stated before, there are many authorities out there, but they do not research and get the correct answers for the RPA issues. Sometimes you may have to do your own leg work to get the information other than the one that your administrators are trying to force feed you. I hope to make every attempt possible to bring you the most up to date information on these matters. There are thirty five states which follow the ARRT testing for RT laws, but the RPA/RA venture is still in its beginning stages. Your individual state department contacts can be found on www.ARRT.ORG . I have provided a table on the next page, to which you may be able to add more information as it becomes available or as the laws as they are passed.

Arkansas-Law-"New and emerging professions" Loophole used for RPA practicing

Colorado- No Law, but very RPA friendly State, Many RPAs Practicing

Georgia- No Law-No problems apparent

Idaho- No Law-At least one RPA

Iowa- Law allowing RPAs to practice will pass may 2005

Kansas- No law-RPA practicing

Kentucky- No Law-RPAs concerned/unable to fluoro and trying to change or add laws

Louisiana- No Law- Practicing RPA

Maryland- Only RT License-One RPA student in the state

Minnesota- No Law- Having difficulty with RPA jobs

Mississippi- 4 RPAs /May have an official amendment for RPA/RA by 7/05

Missouri- No Law, but RPAs think it is needed Practicing RPAs exist

Montana- RPA/RA Law in existence-now defining scope

Nebraska- No Law exists. At least one RPA practicing

Nevada- No current Law, but one may be on the books 2005/2006

New York-"Specialist Assistant" License since 1970/ Granted RPAs to Practice

North Carolina- No RT or RPA laws- RPAs practicing with ease

Oklahoma- No Laws-RPAs practicing with no real problems

Oregon- No Law-"Variance" allows RPAs to do fluoroscopy independent of Radiologist

Pennsylvania- No RT or RPA/RA Law-Many RPAs practicing

Tennessee- Passed Law 7/04- Many RPAs Practicing

Texas- No RPA Law/ RT license allows much RPA scope- Many RPAs practicing

Utah- No laws in place for RPA, but RPAs Practicing with ease

Virginia- No RT or RPA law/ RPAs working but some having problems

Washington- Will confirm Law by 1/05- Many RPAs practicing-May have limited scope

Wyoming- Legislation being drafted right now for the extension of RT license

This data was obtained directly from the RPAs practicing in these states on 11/04. With the ever changing licensure environment of the RPA/RA profession, it is difficult to keep up to date in a book publication. Supplemental information may be available through the RPA/RA programs as it becomes available.

Many Radiology Extenders are having a huge issue with Medicare billing and their levels of supervision. As far as the Medicare patients are concerned, you will have to have personal supervision by the radiologist. This may change in the near future, but it is a restriction at this moment and may be lifted as early as 2005. You can bill under the "incident clause" while working in radiology clinics which are owned by the radiologists themselves or are hospital/radiologist ventures. Look at the compliance requirements for these places, before you agree to perform any procedures on Medicare patients. It would be detrimental to your position, if the salary was based on certain procedures being performed by the RPA and you find out later that you can not bill for them. You can find more information in the CMS guidelines. You may want to review their policies on performing ordered exams and having the ability or not to alter them if needed. I found this information in an Auntminnie article titled, "Medicare Radiology Supervision Rules" by Claudia Murray.

Most radiologists are willing to have the RPA/RA perform as many of the tasks as possible and do the Medicare patients themselves. The radiologists I have spoken with are optimistic that the Medicare levels of supervision can be changed for the Radiologist Extenders in the near future. As the population ages and the Baby boomers require more and more of the radiology services in this country, we won't be able to do without the extenders. There just won't be enough radiologists to go around. We as the first of the RPA/RA types are just ahead of the curve and our patience in this matter will pay off shortly. I still believe that the best way to change the state legislation is to network with the other RPAs/RAs who have drafted legislation in their own states. You can find a copy of the Washington state draft online and some of the other states' as well. Your radiologists should be involved in bringing about this change, at least by helping you get to the right contacts to draft necessary legislation and then of course lending you their utmost support. We should help each other any way we are able.

D.

SETTING UP A PRECEPTORSHIP AND KEEPING IT

Radiology Technologists are not traditionally proposal writers and we don't have to be to achieve this goal. Weber State University has made it easy for us to form an affiliation agreement between the RPA student and the clinical institution. However, to get financial support and a chance for employment once you graduate takes a little bit more. Here is what I did and the suggestions I can give you.

I started with some research which is standard, but I did make a list of things I wanted to accomplish. In order to write a proposal, I needed a general guideline. So, I started with a list which included the following: 1) Write an introduction which will gain the attention of the radiologists as well as the administrators, 2) Show a need for the RPA, 3) Give them the solution to the need which will be fulfilled by the RPA, 4) Help them imagine how the need will be met by having you as the RPA specifically, and 5) you must show what action is needed to fulfill the need you have shown. This will be your intro into the specifics of the RPA negotiations discussed later in the book. Look for my actual proposal in the section about "How to incorporate a Radiologist extender in your radiology practice".

After you have made this outline, you must do the necessary research for each step and keep a journal. This will make the writing process a breeze. For instance, you may want to find out what pains your radiologists have. What bothers them the most about doing their job everyday? Are the problems, time related or money related? You may choose to do some research on what the administrators feel is important. Each situation is different and I can provide some guidance, if needed. You must also do some research on how to present the proposal. It is usually necessary to get a radiologist to sponsor your proposal to be heard by the executive committee of the radiology group.

Cost is another big issue to any company. You must be prepared to discuss and present the monetary implications of your proposal in an itemized form. You may also have to present the details of your preceptorship. This is not so easy since you may be the first RPA student in your practice. Never the less, you should make out a tentative list of what is expected from you and what you expect from your sponsor. Issues like clinical hours paid vs. gratis, scheduling, training, expected productivity and commitment during and after graduation must be considered. You may share and discuss this with your preceptor, but remember to keep a record of these issues. Take notes when you accomplish tasks outlined in the list and when you go above and beyond. You may want to do research on what procedures you are doing and what they bring in for the practice. Cost may be a big issue, but remember that a newly trained radiologist will cost the group at least three to four times what you will be compensated. The radiologists and the administrators know this.

Don't be afraid. If you have done your homework, you will not only get the preceptorship, you will get a free education while being paid for your time. The research you have prepared, will also serve as your guide to maintaining your preceptorship and evaluating your worth to any radiology group. Keep this research handy so that you may use it later in your career. What's more, you may choose to study the section on negotiation before you begin your first semester and lock in your employment. I don't know if this is for everyone, because you do get a different sort of realization after you attend your orientation with the RPA/RA program institution. You will also get a better understanding of what you can offer your respective radiology groups after discussing the changes in laws and strides which have been made between the time period of your application and matriculation.

Example proposal outline at a glance:

1. Introduction
    - Attention getting statistics overworked underpaid radiologists
      i. Trends in health/radiology field

2. Need
    - Justification for RPA/RA existence
      i. Pains discovered at research

3. Solution
    - Satisfactory solution to overworked underpaid radiologists
      i. Any solution you may have found during research

4. How RPA/ RA fills the need
    - Visualization of the RPA taking the load off of the radiologists
      i. Specifics about you and what you can do for them

5. Action/Conclusion
    - Show what specifically must be done now to implement the plan
      i. Cost vs. Benefit along with actions needed
      ii. Don't Forget to include your self the RPA/RA
      iii. Get a lead to the next meeting so you can negotiate further

Some of the RPAs have actually enjoyed the freedom which came from not having a binding employment contract with a radiology group or hospital at the time of matriculation. This left room for negotiation with other radiology groups in the area and a chance to move out of state if they so desired. Having a confirmed contract does however give you a sense of security and alleviates the financial burden while going to school. Along with personal job security you are also giving your radiologist a chance to mold you into the perfect assistant and ensuring continued protection. Since the radiologists have an investment in you, they will try not only to protect it, but will also help you grow. Whichever side you choose, you will at least have the tools and the mindset to proceed.

NOTES (ESSENTIALS AND MY STATE LAWS)

NOTES (ESSENTIALS AND MY STATE LAWS)

CHAPTER 4

DOING WELL IN THE PROGRAM

The first semester-expectations (school, home and work)
How to handle the RTs, supervisors, Radiologists and support staff
The clinicals -What to expect and what to offer
The Hospital vs. Outpatient environment
Difficult subjects: Why learn?

A.

THE FIRST SEMESTER-EXPECTATIONS
(SCHOOL, HOME AND WORK)

My first semester was a fusion of excitement, fear, overwork, familiarity and anticipation which was all very worth it. Of course, everyone has their own touching story and with this thought, I encourage you to look forward to the semester. The staff is wonderful at Weber State, especially when they offer you home baked goods or candy as you enter the radiology department. The teachers are truly inspirational and giving, offering you not only didactic and clinical education, but advice to live your life by. I went to Ogden as a student and came out a student of learning and teaching. I will share with you my strategies for surviving the first semester.

Even though I was a career student with numerous semester hours under my belt, I was amazed at the amount of information we were expected to learn in this first semester. Not to discourage you, but with just the pathophysiology and cross-sectional anatomy being taught by a wonderful, yet very detail oriented lady was enough to make me think twice about goofing off. You will also be learning how to evaluate the osseous system which is very demanding and will be the foundation for everything you do in radiology. Even when you will be doing an UGI or other contrast related procedures, you will be responsible for knowing what boney structures are on the image and what significance the findings have on what you are doing to the patient. My point is that you must make a commitment to work extremely hard not only for the sake of getting through first semester, but to develop an assimilating mind. Integration of all you have learned over the years as great radiographers into the RPA way of thinking will be requisite. You will be considered a mid-level provider and must realize this as such. This first semester will set the tone for the rest of your education.

Specifically you will work with text books as well as supplements called "modules" or other course materials. The Weber program is set up in a way that gives you information that you need to know without you having to buy fifty books. The instructors have taken the areas of importance from several radiology books and after making their own additions have prepared the supplements necessary for your education. Each module will also have your homework assignment and a place to track your grades. This is how you know what is asked of you each time you arrive at the school for your three day session. I made copies of each page and then organized them in the order of the due dates. You can try this or simply make a list of everything that is due in the interim of the two trips. Some of your assignments will be due in between your sessions.

You will have to finish the assignment and either e-mail or snail mail, it to your instructor. Be sure to include the assignment face sheet which is given to you in the beginning of the semester. This is how the teachers track your homework. You will also get your graded homework back when you arrive for your next in school session. Try not to fall behind because you can't build on something you have not learned yet. Sometimes you will be asked to present your homework so that students learn from students. Remember this is about having a good attitude and no one will judge you for your presentation style. The teachers just want to know that you are learning the material needed for the RPA graduation. We had a few shy people, but they learned that it was easier than they had feared. And if presenting is something you enjoy, then this is your chance to get lots of experience. You never know when someone is going to ask you to speak at a conference regarding the RPA/RA issues.

Along with your didactics, you will have to learn how to fit in your new radiology environment. You will be neither an RT nor a Radiologist, and this will create some very strange feelings among your peers and yourself. It all comes down to how you can deal with difficult people. This subject will be covered later in this book, but I do want you to be aware. I felt very alone the first few days of my training and every time I have gone to a different hospital or clinic. Especially after changing jobs and moving out of yet another comfort zone, I had to be prepared for finding a place for my self. The staff really doesn't know what to do with you, because you are not an RT who they can shoot the breeze with. And you are not a radiologist who is being consulted and welcomed by the other physicians. This can make for a difficult situation and I want you to know that you are not alone. It will take time to build rapport with other doctors and the RT staff, but hang in there.

The second semester on the other hand is a breeze compared to the first, didactically speaking. If you keep this in mind you will do great! Remember to keep up with your assigned readings and do the homework! I cannot stress this enough. Students have failed tests, because they underestimated the material. I actually colored the anatomy workbook, took lots of notes when reading and tried to do extra research by asking the radiologists about the areas I did not understand. Some of us bought voice recognition software to help us keep up with the homework and take notes at clinical sites. I found this especially helpful in the first two semesters. Dragon Systems' Naturally Speaking 3.0 Preferred Edition, IBM Via-Voice 98 Executive, L&H Voice X-press Plus, and Philips FreeSpeech98 are some of the systems that are available to you right now. If you want to learn more you can go to http://www.io.com/~hcexres/tcm1603/acchtml/recomx7c.html and find a comparison between all of the voice recognition software listed above. The article is titled, "Voice Recognition Software: Comparison and Recommendations". Even if you don't know anything about computers or voice recognitions programs and you have no idea what I am talking about, this article will help you make the right decision. The article concludes that the Dragon Speak Naturally Speaking was superior overall, but there may be a program that will do what you need it to do for a lot less. Here is what an RPA from Montana had to say. "It's the best $105 I have ever spent" says James Abraham, RPA. He did use the Dragon speak program during his RPA training. On the other hand, I myself used the IBM Via-voice software. It was very inexpensive and did fine after I trained it. This is something you will have to do with any program, no matter which program you choose. Basically you read stories in your own relaxed voice and the program learns how you speak. You might have seen some radiologists use it for dictation. It is quickly becoming the practice for many doctors, not only radiologists.

The next thing to consider is the clinical setting and the procedures expected from you. Although the curriculum does not call for performing fluoroscopic procedures in this first semester, most of your radiologists will insist you cover the fluoroscopic exams which need to be performed in the radiology department. My recommendation is to follow the advice given to you by your teachers, which is based on the curriculum set up for the RPA program. You must try to get a good foundation in pathophysiology, sectional anatomy and bony pathology, before you can effectively perform and understand the reading of the fluoroscopic procedures. When you are performing a fluoroscopic exam, you are not merely taking pictures. Any Technologist can be trained to do that. You are there to be the eyes of the radiologist and although you can't replace the radiologist, you must make every attempt to know what is expected from a radiologist. I actually worked with a group of radiologists who wanted to train their technologists to perform fluoroscopy. It was fine, for a money-saving idea, but not a good one for patient care. Whenever I was in the department observing their work, it lacked the understanding of the human system as a whole. They did not do things systematically and did not know why they should do them in such a way. A perfect example was an esophagram to evaluate the pharynx. The lying down portion was done at the beginning of the exam, and upright lateral swallow was performed at the end. Furthermore, the reason for the exam was, to evaluate for aspiration which had caused pneumonia in this elderly patient. This technologist could not tell me why she should have done the Lateral Swallow in the beginning, or even that she did anything wrong. I can recite examples like this all day long, but the point is; do a service for your patient and don't fall into the trap of being a "picture taker".

Another great reason for waiting to perform these fluoroscopic procedures is that, when you actually do start performing the procedures, you will have little time to learn much of anything else. You will be expected to keep a schedule and take care of what a RPA on staff would normally do. Take it from me, I have been there. I had no children to tend to so I had the extra time needed to learn other things which should have been taken care of during the eight hour clinical time. Ultimately, the choice is yours.

Let me leave you with one more thought on this subject. Be aware of your limitations. Look at your curriculum and practice in clinicals, what you are learning in the classroom. You do have the freedom to be flexible, because this is not a traditional classroom type program, but be careful. After all, a lab is supposed to be used as a means to reinforce what you learned in the didactic arena. Please don't be scared into doing things you do not want to do, because when things go wrong, your preceptors will go by the curriculum and its limitations. Remember, you won't loose your preceptorship for not performing what is not in the curriculum, but you will loose it for doing too much, too soon, whether you cause harm to the patient or not there will be negative consequences. This vary thing happened to me. I was able to salvage this because I stuck to the curriculum, but I did have to fight the radiologists all the way. They wanted me to perform exams which had not been covered in the syllabus as of yet and so I refused. Even if you are going by the rules, there can be some gray areas.

I was just about to graduate, when I was called upon to perform a Thyroid biopsy. I had consulted with two other radiologists, one of whom was the chief of radiology. I thought I was doing a great thing, because, I was saving them time. Thyroid biopsies can be time consuming, if you don't know this by now. Little did I know that I was supposed to have personal supervision for this procedure, I had performed it many times on my own and gotten very good at it. Well, I was performing this on a nurse who had wanted the Chief of Radiology to perform the procedure. I went through all of the necessary steps from obtaining consent to saying good bye after a very successful biopsy confirmed by the pathologist. Well, to my surprise, I was now being reprimanded for not having a radiologist in the room and being accused of practicing medicine without a license. This was absurd. I had all of the legal paperwork and the curriculum from the school. On the agreement it was clearly stated that if I proved my competency for performing a certain task, that I in fact did not need a physician present in the room. These things saved me and I was doing things by the book. The patient was not ill treated and the procedure was executed flawlessly. Yet, my right to be considered for full privileges at that hospital came to a halt. I could not obtain any privileges in any of the hospitals in that system. It was such a waste. This was only due to miscommunication between the chief of radiology and the chief medical staff officer. You can only imagine what would have happened to me and my career if I was doing anything remotely outside of what the curriculum dictated at that time. I don't intend to scare you into being a chicken, but don't be a liability either. Have a good communication system with your radiologists. It is alright to question them and make sure you do things by the book, even if it means having the patient wait a few more minutes.

It is difficult to corner a doctor for any advice let alone educational guidance, but you must be willing to give it a good try. Whether it is a procedure related question or didactics, most radiologists do remember they were residents once. If they don't remember, just remind them. You just have to find the radiologists to help you. Possessing a positive attitude and without appearing confrontational will give you the best way to get in with the radiologist. Even if the radiologist has been giving you the run around and not answering your questions, it's a good idea to keep smiling. If this totally fails, use the web sites and make sure you understand the material. When you have more information about the topic in question; then you can approach the radiologists one more time. When you can communicate with them on their own level, they may respond better. Another resource to consider is the instructor who is teaching the class which covers the topic you have questions about. Don't be shy, all of the instructors are eager to help you learn. If you have tried everything, keep in touch with the other RPA students, and we can all work together to help you. There is a group session for the Weber State RPA students and you can get some help there. I had a few close friends who were RPA students and we exchanged e-mails and kept in touch that way. The teachers don't mind this as long as you don't take the tests together. And as always, it would be my pleasure help you, in any way that I can.

During this first semester is when most people will have doubts about their abilities as students and as functioning RPAs. We all need a little something to keep us going at this time. I had a lot of uncertainty, which passed as the semester progressed. My uneasiness ranged from, fitting in to feeling comfortable with more responsibility when it comes to patient care. By finishing all of my homework on time for the classes I was rewarded by being able to participate in the class discussions. You just have to trust me on this one, you will feel it too. When you are well prepared for the three day trip to school, the confidence just radiates from within you. The teachers help will build your confidence and give you advice on the latest laws and trends which involve the RPA profession. Before you know it, you will be finishing the semester and moving on to more advanced clinical learning and the second semester. Moreover, you will begin to appreciate yourself for getting through some of these hurdles.

Now, don't forget to have some fun. I found camaraderie to be essential in a new field that is just getting started. Ogden has great places to ski and wonderful restaurants to dine. We as students would get together at one of the themed restaurants and learn more about each other. Some restaurants were very romantic and when we brought our significant others along for the winter trips, it was heavenly. I hope you will enjoy your trips as much as I did. Look inside your "Everything you wanted to know about Ogden, Utah, But were afraid to ask…" booklet. This will be given to you from the school. It contains everything you should need to get around the area, and have lots of fun! For students attending other programs, don't just study the whole time. Have your homework assignments done so that you may enjoy the surrounding landscape and your new friends.

B.

How to handle the RTs, supervisors, Radiologists and support staff

It is always difficult to be the so called "trail blazer". Having heard this so many times throughout my schooling, I began to hate the expression. It is very true though. We are paving our own way. We have the guidance and the resources, but we must make our own road and then walk on it, whether it is fast or slow. Many obstacles will be present at your work place and even in your social circles. These hurdles are beginning to dissipate as the acceptance of the RPA/RA grows. Never the less, you must be prepared to handle them in a delicate manner. Try not to burn any bridges by antagonizing or alienating the radiology nurses and your fellow technologists or better yet the other mid-level providers. I would suggest that you find a good book which talks about how to handle difficult situations and use it as a guide. I will try to touch on this, but the subject has so many facets and the specialist to cover them, that I will not be that detailed. This is based exclusively on my experiences and you should take them as such.

You will have a tremendous knowledge base, not only in radiology, but in general which will only grow during your career. It is easy to let this new found advantage over your surrounding co-workers have a negative impact. Your humble beginnings are easily forgotten as the new found knowledge and prestige take over your psyche. You must try to remember where you came from and if done in a constructive manner, you can help the people around you feel more comfortable with you. By including them in the patient care and decision making process and teaching them about things you wondered about when you were in their place can make for a smooth transition. While doing all of this, don't seem too desperate to make friends either. While you are teaching, don't forget to learn and give credit where it's due. Being nice to just one nurse or technologist can set a precedence of acceptance. We are not doctors and it is good if we can remember this. We are trying to bridge the gap between the radiologist and the technological and nursing staff. This will be difficult to do if you are not working as a team. Once you get this across to the team, including your self, you will have no trouble with staff conflicts. Some people will not want to be your friends and that's alright. They might have some insecurity issues that only a psychologist can address. It's not your place and you should not let this discourage you. You have worked hard and are trying to be sensitive to the staff and others in your environment. There is nothing else you can do. As long as you can get most of the team to be a cohesive unit, you can get along with most other disapproving persons.

However, I did find that the when I rotated through the different facilities, the people who were strangers turned out to be the nicest, to me. I worked in a set of outpatient radiology clinics and knew most of the people working there. At one office, everyone who was not at the management level was wonderful. The manager however tried to diminish my accomplishments and voiced her own stories of being a very talented technologist in the seventies who already knew all of things I was being trained to do. Later I discovered that she felt a little threatened and lost. People in her position often feel that they just did so much for the radiologists and now another person was going to come in and invade their little close knit family. After all the managers would like to think they are the favorites of the Radiologists. Now they knew that I was closer to the radiologists and threatened the delicate relationships they had formed. The personal conversations they were used to having with the doctors were quickly vanishing as they gave me more and more of their attention. I guess you can equate it to kind of a second child syndrome. Where the older child starts throwing fits and begins misbehaving to get more attention from the parents as they are busy nurturing the younger sibling. This is the kind of behavior I have seen. Your experiences will vary, but try not to look past these issues. Some people try to ignore them, but addressing them is a better decision.

Some of the managers didn't even know anything about the RPA position and wanted to rebel against the Radiologists for tossing them to me. Communication can play a big role in any situation, especially with the introduction of not only a new person, but a totally new profession. To overcome the awkwardness of being in this situation, take these few steps. This may or may not work, but at least you will have tried. First, define your position and get it in writing. Second, have the company newsletter post your position and your general responsibilities. If you don't have a newsletter, you can have a memorandum sent out by the appropriate persons to the appropriate parties. Finally, when you go to a new facility, meet the manager and have them introduce you to the staff. You should try and have a meeting with the manager before hand so that you can go over what your and the manager's expectations are. After you both are on the right page, the manager should address the staff and present them with your level of authority. This will ensure that you get the proper staff compliance and the respect that comes with working as a team. This is what went wrong with my introduction to my former company.

If I myself, had followed the steps listed above, I am certain the outcome of my experience, would have been more favorable. You don't want to wind up in a position where the staff is barking orders at you and treating you as if you are a technologist there to help them. This can happen and has happened to even some radiologists I have known. Can you believe that the technological staff tried to get a radiologist to do portables in the emergency room, because they did not know who he was? It happened and it was easily correctable, because they knew what a radiologist's job description is. We do not have a clear cut job description. Most people in the medical community don't even know we exist, let alone what our role encompasses. The job description will most definitely vary according to your facility and your contract. More importantly, neither the technological staff nor the management team will have much idea of what your capabilities or credentials are. So, it will be up to you to set the stage for what you want out of the workday. On the first day, take your credentials with you and leave a copy with the management. Also, bring along your logs or an excel spread sheet of all of the procedures you have ability to perform. You may want to get one of the radiologists to sign the excel spread sheet as well. I actually take a couple of magazines that have featured the RPA/RAs in them and leave them for the staff to read. They are curious about you, but they don't want to ask. After they read the articles, they are more likely to approach you. I have had a great amount of success with this and let me tell you. I know of several technologists who are applying to the RPA program, because of me. This is the best compliment; I could ever hope to receive.

In other settings, you may have a manager, who thinks you can do more than your scope of practice dictates. This happened to me at the offices where the management personnel were not promoted from a technologist position to a manager's level. They were chosen mainly for their leadership abilities and organizational skills. This is happening all over the medical practice, where it is not a pre-requisite to be medical personnel, before being offered management status at a medical facility. In this case, you should educate the manager about your limitations and job duties. I found that these managers were very receptive and gave me much deserved respect. They wanted to learn some of the technical and medical aspects of radiology from me and even involved me with staff issues, patient management and technical decisions in their office or department. They conveyed to me that they could see the tremendous potential of the RPA position, only after they understood it. So, things can vary with personalities, management backgrounds, and the familiarity of the persons with you and the RPA profession.

When I was in the hospital setting, I received praise for being the first RPA student and the technologists wanted to know how they could get involved and learn to do what I was doing. This was such a change from the radiology clinics owned by my group. I had to treat the hospital management much like the ignorant child, because I was a stranger in their radiology department and they would need to know and be responsible for my actions. I was not their employee and I did not know their policies. It is a good idea to meet with the manager, director and the chief of radiology to discuss the legal implications of having an RPA or a RPA student in the department. What orientation classes I needed to attend or paperwork I needed to file. You may have taken care of this in your preceptorship and affiliation agreement, but it doesn't hurt to have the meeting and go through all of this again. Make sure the manager and the radiologist introduce you to the staff while informing them of your abilities, authority and limitations. I can not stress this enough. This is what made my experience so very pleasant at the hospitals.

My philosophy is that if you can swing it, do your preceptorship away from the technologists that you already know and work with. You will learn a lot more when you are not constantly facing contempt. If you can't change your destiny, then try this. Be very polite and offer to help the management as much as you can. Even if you have to spend a little bit of your own time, it will be worth it. Try teaching the technologists and the managers, new techniques that are coming out and try to say that they would be great at being an RPA if they had the chance. Give them some respect if you want to receive it yourself. If you plan to stay with your present company, you have to make this work. This is because after you graduate, these managers will be the ones to get you through your day with ease. They control the staff and they will ultimately control your time as well. You must do some research to find out what role will they play in your career after you have graduated.

In smaller companies you may have no trouble with this issue, but in my case it was no small task. In a large radiology group with hundreds of employees and a large management staff, it is a very political game. Unless they see a clear advantage, the top directors will not want to help you, especially, if you are getting along so very nicely with the radiologists. I failed to play by their rules. They wanted me to train technologists to perform the tasks of the RPA, just because there were no laws stopping it. It was ethically and professionally wrong and I did not do it. For this I was put in a position to work under management instead of being a medical staff person, like the radiologists had wanted. They also, trained these so called "fluoro techs", even though the sole reason that the ACR stepped in with the RPA issue was to stop such antics. You may fail to see that the radiologists are very busy and that is why they hire people to take care of their businesses. So, they do not have much control of your destiny, unless it has to do with procedures at the hospital. Please, think twice about the type of situation you want to be in and do your homework. I have found that a small practice may be the right niche for the RPA. As you can see, either you can pave a bright future for you, or shoot your self in the foot, or both can happen. I have tried a large group and now I am giving a small startup group a chance. If you do your own research, you can locate just the right environment for you. You may have to wait for the right one to come along, but you should not settle, just because you need a job today. Start early, at least 6-8mos in advance and you won't be in that predicament.

C.

THE CLINICALS
WHAT TO EXPECT AND WHAT TO OFFER

Most radiologists are afraid to train a RPA student at first. They have mixed feelings about the concept and insecurities of their own profession. Most radiologist groups have a governing committee and they may be the ones who agreed to your training. The problem is that the poor radiologist who has been designated to train you has reservations. They don't want to go against the wishes of the group, yet they don't want to accept you as a student. What do you do? Here's what I did.

I was actually put in this situation. We had over fifty radiologists and the one who sponsored me was not the one assigned to train me. This was good and bad. It was very beneficial to learn every aspect of radiology from the person who was fellowship trained in that sub-specialty. However, some radiologists don't get along with others and when they know that you are [their] project they don't want to teach you. Well, I started out learning from a radiologist who was in pediatrics. I had never worked with him or at this hospital. I was assigned to the ER board reading room (Before PACS) at this trauma center. I was seeing so many modalities and pathology that I went home with a tremendous tension headache. I didn't ever get headaches, so I was really concerned. My headaches lasted for about one month and then they disappeared. This may happen to you if you are being overloaded with information and you try to learn it all in one day. Try to take breaks, even if it means missing out on a cool case. You will learn more efficiently with the break system. Once I learned this, I felt better too. Sometimes I would fall into my old habit and pay for it later with a headache. The US Army gave me an ulcer and now I was getting headaches; what a trade off.

Well, I gave it my all in the first few months and it paid off. The pediatric radiologist not only taught me adult radiology, but he encouraged me to learn pediatrics. I truly lucked out! Two months into the program after hearing how well I was doing, the interventional radiologist who was also the chief of the radiology department at the hospital, decided that he was going to give me a chance. I tried to be humble, but affirmed. I learned to show what I knew by asking questions rather than finding fault with what the radiologist had read. When I knew something was being missed on the film, I would ask a question about the pathology instead of saying that something was being missed. You do not want to insult your teachers no matter what's being missed on the film. You don't have to try and prove that you know more then them. Don't do this! I followed the question method, until we (radiologist and I) became comfortable with each other. Now we are truly good friends and have tremendous respect for one another. The older radiologists may or may not accept you at first and you have to feel this out for your self. Once I graduated, I found that the older radiologists really appreciated me and my skills. They would even start telling me stories about how a long time ago they used to take images and then trained the technologists to do them. Also, they informed me that they had trained technologists to perform some of the tasks the RPAs are doing now. But in the olden days, the techs just learned on the job and the radiologists were comfortable with them. I would have to say that most of the radiologists you encounter will treat you with respect if you earn it.

The moral of this is that you should make do with what you have, learn what you can and apply it to your advantage when the opportunity presents itself. If you can't learn from people, use books or other means. Keep expanding your mind because you will need it. Find out when and where all of the hospital conferences are being held. You may want to find Mammo, GI, Cancer and trauma conferences to name a few. These will help you learn and to get you some CMEs. The extra bonus will come from meeting the doctors and the residents who will also be attending. I attended a teaching session for the internal medicine residents, trauma conferences and cancer treatment sessions which proved invaluable to me.

On the matter of clinical hours and how to satisfy them: Well, the school requires that you spend at least eight hours per week reading films with a radiologist. It is further required that you get 16-24 hours of hands on clinical training time. This can be accomplished by either working on the weekends and having clinicals during the week or working during the week and doing the clinicals on the weekends. Radiologists do not want to spend any extra time in the hospitals on the weekends, but you can hang out and read films with them for that requisite. Maybe you can offer to do the minor fluoroscopy procedures for them in return. Take notes on things you don't understand and look them up in Paul and Juhl's text book. You will need to keep this one handy as well as some of the others your teachers will recommend. You can try it one way or the other and do what is right for you, but before you decide to give up, talk to the teachers and get their advice. Do not quit! You will probably regret it in the end. My RPA training passed so quickly, that I know if I would have second guessed my self, I would have regretted it. I am more financially stable and feel more satisfied with my career. You too deserve the acknowledgement for what you know and have achieved.

Some students think that they have to stick to one preceptor for every aspect of the clinicals. The fact of the matter is you should get the best part of your training from whoever is willing to give it to you. If you are friends with a radiologist and he is willing to let you hang out and read films, then do it. You can work with the school to get everything worked out. You may have to have 2 or even 3 affiliation agreements signed, but you will get through your clinicals. You may have one radiologist who works at one hospital and he is willing to teach you angiography, yet you have another who is willing to show you general fluoroscopy and minor invasive procedures. You have to give your self a chance to learn from both. Most students are lucky enough to get everything at one academic environment, but some are not. There were some students in the earlier classes who had to go to nearby states to get someone to let them perform certain procedures for requisite. That's what I call resourcefulness. You don't have to be that creative, but you may have days when you are not getting to as much as you should.

I have discovered that some schools will be offering preceptorships as part of their package. This will alleviate the need for extra work on the student's part. One such school is University of Medicine and Dentistry in New Jersey. They do however; require you to possess a bachelor's degree with a 3.0GPA, have three years of radiologic technologist experience, a New Jersey state license and/or ARRT certification and ACLS completion. The choices will be there for you, but you will have to do some homework. It's actually a good idea to have some of the medical schools teach the RA and RPA curricula. This will give us the notoriety we will need to be widely accepted within the medical community. Once you have secured a program and a preceptorship, you will get a chance to learn the procedures.

On the actual procedures at hand, first figure out what your strong areas will be. For example, if you are a sonographer, you may want to try doing Paracenthesis or Thoracenthesis. If you are an angiographer, you may want to try a femoral stick and moving the catheter down for an aorta runoff etc… Work with what you know first. Not only will this build your confidence, but it will help the radiologist see how useful you can be. If you can take over some of the tasks which are time consuming for the radiologist, they will use that time to teach you. If they don't see this trade off, you can keep track of the time you have saved, in a journal. Later, use this to ask for some student question answer time. You can't just ask for stuff, you have to earn it. While trying to save the radiologist time, I hope you will not fall into a common pitfall. We like to help the doctors. This is what drives us as auxiliary personnel. The one thing we don't want to do is jeopardize our training and preceptorship with a facility. So remember, don't ever try to do more than you are trained to do and what you and your radiologist <u>both</u> feel comfortable with. If you don't follow this, you will have a short lived career. Try to follow the clinical book schedule, but don't let it bind you either. Learn as much as you can while practicing good common sense.

I wanted to touch on the legal issues of a preceptorship for a moment. Please read the affiliate agreement carefully and follow it to the letter. Make sure you have a legal agreement with the hospital where you are training as well as the radiology group. Your radiologists may or may not know or tell you what is needed in each case. It is your responsibility to go to the medical staffing office and let them know what you are trying to accomplish. I would try doing this a few months before your clinicals begin. Most hospitals require you to have personal supervision for most procedures and they do not care about the school policy that says we can do procedures on our own once we have been deemed competent. This means that the radiologist <u>must</u> be in the room when you perform the procedure! Try if you can to set up something in the contract that states you can have three supervised procedures and then be able to perform them without the radiologist physically in the room. Be very careful with the language and this will keep you from loosing your chance at hospital privileges after you graduate. Remember for most of the states, the RPAs and students are working under the "Delegation" clause. Also, keep in mind that Medicare patients cannot be billed if the radiologist does not provide personal supervision. Keep a log of all of the procedures you observe, perform or assist in. make sure you get informed consent for every procedure you perform and keep a copy for your self. This will serve as your record of competency for future credentialing processes. If you work for the hospital, have a copy of these logs placed in your permanent file as well.

For some of us who need a more structured approach to radiology practice, I recommend that you go to www.auntminnie.com and download the guide to residency in diagnostic radiology. You can use this as a means to check yourself in the clinical setting. Also, you can use this to gage what you are learning compared to what a radiology resident is required to know. I found this very helpful and hope you will too. You should be set for your clinical experience now.

D.

The Hospital vs. Outpatient environment

No matter which environment you encounter you have to learn to adjust. If you are in an outpatient clinic, you may not have the dreaded credentialing issues, but you may not be able to satisfy all of your clinical requirements. In some situations, your supervisors may ask you to perform technologist duties which will prevent you from having adequate time for RPA work. It is easy to get caught up in this so, set your boundaries before your clinicals begin. Have a meeting with your supervisor, director and the radiologist who is the preceptor. Set some guidelines and get them in writing. You may encounter that they promise to get it in writing and you never get it. Write down your expectations of the guidelines and have them signed off by the attending parties. This way you have a record of what is expected. You may want to set the mornings for tech work and afternoons for RPA, but you must do it.

Please don't fall into the trap of doing tech work in the RPA time if you see that your friends are busy. We all like to help, especially if you are a good tech and you fear loosing your friends. If they are truly your friends they will understand. After all, this is your time and you need to fulfill your new job duties which are now different than the ones before. So if you view it as you are doing your new job, then it may make it easier to let the busy people do the imaging while you sit by the radiologist and observe. This was very difficult for me when I was at some of the outpatient clinics where I worked as a tech before enrolling in the RPA program. You may have to take some of your co-workers aside and let them know that it may look unfair that I am sitting reading films with the radiologist while they are running around crazy. Let them know that if you are doing your new job now and if you don't pass your tests, you will fail in your new job duties. They will understand and will even try to help you by showing you cool cases.

Even if you get all of this in a harmonious order, you may not be able to satisfy your procedural requirements at an outpatient site. This is why it is a good idea to have an agreement with a hospital as well. Consult this book, talk to your radiologist about what you are lacking and find a hospital that will grant you preceptorship. You can do this even if you didn't do it before starting the clinicals.

The hospital setting provides you with a wealth of knowledge, but it comes with the price of dealing with the medical staffing office. Just like you had to appeal to the radiology group, now you must make your case to the medical executive committee of the hospital. This is not so easy, since your radiologists don't want you to be a part of it. They want to deal with it with a handshake. Don't let them do this. You must try and convince them that all legal issues have to be addressed so that you don't terminate your own career. The hospitals will need to know about your governing body and who is responsible for you. Remember we are governed by the Certification board of Radiology Practitioner Assistants (CBRPA). Further we must report to the ARRT and the state health department if your state has RT/RPA/RA license regulations. If you look at it, we function much like the sonographers and as the sonographers have the ARDMS, we have the CBRPA. Neither one of us have the ARRT's testing requirement. The ARDMS had existed for a long time until the ARRT decided they too were going to offer the sonography examinations. Now the ARRT is offering the RA testing for the 2005 graduates, mainly so that they can have a quicker start than they did with the sonographers' testing. On a brighter note, the hospital staff will be more receptive towards you than the outpatient clinic.

For legal responsibility issues, refer to the nurses, paramedics, technologists and other physician extenders for whom the doctors are ultimately responsible. Whether it is an outpatient or a hospital facility, the doctors are responsible for more than they would like to admit to. Remind them that we do carry our own liability insurance through the school. This will help speed things along. The first thing you will need is the HIPPA form filled out and signed by you, so that you can at least observe the pathologies that are unique to the hospital setting. While you are waiting for the credentialing approval to be granted, you can learn the workflow of the radiology department, policy and procedures and feel comfortable with your new environment. This way when you do get the privileges to perform procedures you won't be estranged. How do you expect to make the patients comfortable, when you are not yourself? So, even if it takes months to get credentialing, do not despair. Use your time for other learning experiences. I was in the middle of my clinicals when I discovered more paperwork had to be filed and that paperwork would take three months to get approved. I was shocked and felt as if my RPA career had come to an end. I looked at all of my options and used my time to observe more complicated procedures, learn to understand more imaging modalities, and performed preliminary reading on all images on the reading boards. I would not have had the chance to do this if I was doing fluoroscopy all day and having a few hours a day to learn imaging pathology. I feel I am a better RPA toady because of that setback.

E.

DIFFICULT SUBJECTS: WHY LEARN?

With any course of study you will encounter subjects which are easy to comprehend and some you wish had just been hard wired into your brain. I will discuss some of the topics which may be difficult, yet necessary. Learning to think in three dimensions in cross sectional anatomy, the science of cells with regards to pathophysiology, radiation physics and new clinical language and skills can be extremely demanding. Some subject areas seem important at first glance and don't need further persuasion to it's necessity. Having an understanding of how the subject matter will affect your practice will help you deal with this in a more reasonable manner.

For example, the medical terminology which is used commonly by the physicians is a crucial part of being a physician extender. We must learn to speak the language, yet I find that most of us don't. If we can't understand the orders and the patient's condition which may be written by the physician or being discussed in the hallway, we are at a disadvantage. Having information will always give you an edge in deciding what action should be taken in any scenario. You may be getting ready to perform a diagnostic procedure during which you are to locate the source of the person's said problem. If you do not know what that problem is, because it is in some medical jargon, you will be at an obvious disadvantage. Having been in this position myself, I would recommend that you get your self a good medical terminology book and add it as a supplement to your studies. You should practice using the medical language rather than resorting back to the layman's terms. Don't get me wrong, you still have to explain it to the patients in common language, but when you are talking with the staff and the physicians, use the medical jargon. Once you have this taken care of, you can start with the RPA/RA curriculum.

The one thing I can not stress enough is to do your homework. No matter how tedious it may seem. There were times when I thought I was going to pass out with my face in the pathophysiology book. I may have fallen asleep at times, but no major medical damage. Next, do all of the pre-tests that are in the course materials and keep them handy. You will also get a chance to work on-line with your classmates on cases. You should take this opportunity to expand your mind and learn about the medical aspects of the patient, which will prove very helpful in clinicals. This was a chance for me to learn about different medical conditions which can present in an imaging environment and how to form a clinical pathway for it. Next, keep "Paul and Juhl's" handy along with the pathophysiology and sectional anatomy books. You may want to take them to clinicals with you. "Paul and Juhl's" has all basic radiology imaging and processes. You can reference practically any thing you need during the day. The only problem is that it weighs a lot!

If you want, you may want to also add "Squire's Fundamentals of Radiology" to your list as well. This book is a little bit lighter. As a matter of fact some of my radiologists had mentioned that if I just studied the Squire's book, I could be a radiologist. There are also small books called "the requisites". These books are divided by category and you can pick the category you are studying at the time and take the book with you to clinicals. If you are attending the WSU program I would definitely take the current clinical subject modules with you.

You can take your pick, but don't forget to study everything you have. This was my mistake. I kind of forgot about the Squire's book and then had to go back and re-learn some of the basics. Having good resources will prove very valuable to you. I say this because, depending on the facility and the radiologist, you may not have many reference books or they may be out dated. For anatomical references having outdated books is not such a big deal, since the human body has not changed much, but for imaging this is big. New modalities and ways to look at pathology have made it difficult to keep up with the new books and journals. Never the less, we must try to keep up with our required texts and this will get us through most of the clinicals. Later in your own practice you may want to subscribe to new books and journals being offered in your specialty. Being a member of some of the radiologist societies will get you some of the publications, but don't hold your breath. I tried to join a few of these societies and was denied. We are making strides and the ARRS has made a place for us.

I have found that having the most recent material is great, but having at least the RPA program texts were enough to get me through training. I keep at least a $500 budget to spend on resources every year for my continuing RPA education. This is only for texts and journal subscriptions. You may want to spend less. It just depends on how much time you have to read and what your work library consists of. The pathophysiology book is great too, especially for its clinical lab values. I would recommend just making a copy of pertinent areas and carrying that with you, because the book will take your arm off, if you try to take it every where with you. If you work in the Interventional suite you could possibly store it there, if it's secure. You don't want to have to buy another one. They are not cheap either.

Here are the subjects that I see as challenges, not because they are difficult, but because it is easy to breeze past them without spending the adequate time needed to fully appreciate the material for its application and necessity. The RPA program is very intense, but I do hope that you spend a little extra time on the courses listed below.

Evaluating the Osseous System:

This course can be easy as well as challenging. Bones are the most apparent images of the body when thinking about imaging. Since you can visualize boney anatomy virtually in any procedure that you are performing, this makes it even more important. You are now going to be the eyes of the radiologist and must see all of the findings, whether they are related to the procedure at hand or not. Learning and retaining the information about boney pathology is imperative. Most people think they already know what they are seeing on a skeletal image. This can make this a silent learning challenge, because most radiologic technologists feel very comforted in their ability to diagnose bony processes. After all they have been doing it for years and years; diagnosing for the nurses and the Emergency room physicians. Don't neglect this course and be duped into making common mistakes, which can make you look incompetent.

Psycho-Social Medicine:

This course can be a bit tricky to you in an unusual way. The majority of us have to deal with very sick people in varying situations. Knowing how to deal with a diversified patient population with varying cultures and beliefs is the key to avoiding most problems. Let's say you have a person who is very suspecting and is not offering any medical history. It is becoming very difficult for you to assess the medical condition and or contraindications for the procedure you are trying to perform. If you knew why they were doing this, then you can come up with ways to persuade the patient to help you. Studying different population groups and integrating their commonalities and differences can lead to better communication between you and the patient. According to the article published in Radiology Today in the September/ October issue of 2004, "Legal Trends in Radiology," "Numerous malpractice suits are based on a lack of communication between care providers and patients and between care providers themselves".

Medical Ethics and Law:

After reading the above mentioned article as a directed reading from the ASRT, I realized why we need to know and understand the laws that affect us as Radiologic Technologists and as Radiologist Extenders. With such a new field you have to make it a priority to know what pertains to you and learn how to decipher the legal issues. You are ultimately responsible for your actions. I discovered this during my training as an RPA and have made it my number one priority to know more about the legalities of every situation and protocol I am directly involved in. This course gives you an appreciation for ethical dilemmas and the legalities which bind us.

All of the other courses are needed to fulfill the clinical aspect of your training and you are less likely to forget about them. I just wanted to focus on the ones you may consider a nuisance, rather than a necessity. Let me assure you that you will need these courses and you will use them.

NOTES (SCHOOL AND CLINICALS)

CHAPTER 5
SECURING EMPLOYMENT

When and how to negotiate an employment contract
Professionalism and attitude becoming a RPA/RA
Hospital credentialing after you graduate
How to put together a credentialing form

A.

When and how to negotiate an employment contract

After all of your hard work it would be nice to have a satisfying career with just rewards. You must have a plan of action, whether you have a contract or not. If you already have a contractual agreement with your preceptor and have a satisfying quid pro quo, then you are probably alright. If you do not have a contract or an offer letter by the time you are six months away from graduation, you have to get on the ball.

Remember all of the research I asked you to do in chapter 3, section d? You will need it now. Follow the steps below and you too may have an agreeable outcome:

1. Gather all of your research (needs of doctors, administrators, budgets etc...)

2. Set a goal for your self (what is important? Money, location, time)

3. Follow steps in chapter 3 and form a general guideline for a proposal

4. Get a meeting with the radiology group and/or the CEO of the company

Step four is difficult, but it shouldn't be too tough if you have been speaking with the important decision makers during your RPA training. Make sure you know who the decision makers are. You don't want to waste time and effort on someone who does not have the authority to either take your offer to the decision makers, nor is the decision maker themselves. Finding the right job is essential since you are a rarity. Remember you can save the radiology group a lot of money and partnership quarrels. This is not to say that you shouldn't ask for a partnership track. You should ask for anything and everything you wish to gain out of the deal. If you don't put it on the table, you will never know if this was indeed in their budget. You can always come down from what you are asking, but it's difficult to demand more at a later date. It is also complicated to get raises when you are already a part of the team. Don't forget, it is hard to hire radiologists right now. Keep all of this in mind and contact the person who is going to get you in. Sometimes it's even the CEO's assistant. Gather current data on what their needs are and what possible solutions they have looked at. Find out where they stand on RPAs. After concluding your research and forming a guideline, you should write your proposal. There are many books available and web sites you can use. I was able to type in "proposal writing" into Google search at www.google.com and get many hits. If you would like to contact me, I can give you more guidance in this matter.

After you have a written proposal, set up the meeting to discuss this matter. You may what to do a little check list to brainstorm any questions or concerns the meeting may bring up. You should have pre-emptive responses for these. If something does come up and you do not know what you should say, just tell them you need to research it and you will get back to them. Then make a list of the items and follow through on the research. You will make a good impression if you do this. Do not be intimidated in the meeting. No one has all of the answers to everything and if you act like you do, then you may even leave a negative impression.

If you get the meeting with a group you have already been working for, you are lucky. In this case, go ahead and have the meeting. Stay on track and address every important issue. Important issue that is important to both parties not just to you. Try to think of the other person across the desk. This will keep you out of trouble. If they are interested, ask for another meeting. The next meeting can be used to talk about the actual details of employment and to ask for a written offer letter or contract. Don't do anything with a handshake. You might get too excited, because they are giving you more than you could have ever imagined, but get it in writing! I have been burned by this and it is not something you want to experience. So, I will say it again; get the conditions and benefits of your employment contract in writing!

If you are like the many RPAs out there who are venturing out to find employment with groups who they know only by name and reputation, this is for you. Before you set up a meeting to discuss your future with a group, you must prepare a Powerpoint presentation or something similar to showcase your position. Even if they don't want you to present, it is a good idea to let them know you did prepare one. My experience has taught me that employers will eventually want to see what you can do for the company, mainly to see the cost vs. benefit ratio. A Power-Point presentation can be very supportive of you and a precursor to more opportunities. This presentation should highlight the RPA/RA as a benefit, but you should also discuss other issues. There should be an introduction, trends, laws, salary, and specifically how an RPA/RA can help their practice. Think in their world, not what you want. You will have time for this a little later. If you have this handy, then you can ask the CEO to have a small meeting with you to discuss a new option for them in terms of the manpower crisis. From here you can go into the steps listed above. In chapter 8, you will find some examples which may be helpful.

This takes much commitment, but it does pay off. As the RPAs/RAs become more affluent in our society, you will have to do less Powerpoint and more negotiating. It is not a bad idea to get some books on negotiating and read them after you graduate. Yes, they are a Google search away. Negotiation tactics and how to utilize them effectively is an asset to anyone who is involved in contract relationships. Whether you stay with the preceptor group or venture out, you can benefit by learning how to negotiate. Which brings me to the Radiologist Extenders, who may or may not want to stay with the same group with whom they gained clinical experience?

The RPAs who want to be locked into a contract before starting school will have to do the research and follow the guidelines 1-4 above. The only difference is that you want to leave the contract a little loose. By this I mean you may want to give your self an "out" if needed. I am not saying to use trickery, not that the company lawyers will let you. You do not know what the salary range for your skill level will be in two years, so ask for a range rather than a fixed figure. Try to list the kinds of services you will be proving for such a salary. This way if they promise you $75K to do just fluoroscopy and later their needs change and you are asked to perform invasive procedures as well, then you should be able to say the salary range for this skill is $30K more than the fluoroscopist, which is listed in the contract. New contract should be drawn up and executed per the desired skill set they would like you to utilize. Some people like fixed amounts and if you are conservative in this manner, there is nothing wrong with a flat amount, as long as you have a good idea of what your procedure load and difficulty and legal risk level will encompass.

Hopefully you can see how easy it is to get duped into doing more for less. You are one of the front runners in this race, don't get left behind. You must push the envelope and strive to get as much as you can which shows your importance to the medical community. I am not saying you should be greedy, but you should ask for what is considered "fair market value". Unfortunately, the "fair market value" will keep fluctuating until we have enough RPA/RAs to meet the demand. Geographical regions and the radiology practices dictate the going rate, so be conscientious of changes. Look over the expansion plans of the radiology group and or company you are considering, as well as the radiologist extender scope of practice. You as a RPA/RA should know more about your profession, than anyone who is not.

B.

PROFESSIONALISM AND ATTITUDE BECOMING A RPA/RA

Now that you have landed your self a job as a true physician extender, you must learn to act like one. It is easy to fall back into your old habits of being a technologist as I am speaking from personal experience. It is ok to keep your assets, but you try not to incorporate any bad habits. We are an extension of the radiologist, and thus we should be a good representation of that radiologist and his/her group. We should try to set our differences aside when it comes to competing professions and embrace the philosophy that everyone has a role to play and everyone can be an asset to the radiology department.

Starting from your physical appearance to the mind set, you must always appear confident, but not arrogant. Even if the radiologists may sometimes appear that way themselves. Clothing should be professional at all times when in the workplace. Some people say that your appearance should reflect where you want your career to go, at all times of the day, not just in a work place setting. You may have heard about "dressing for success". When I was an independent "Mary Kay" consultant, we were encouraged to wear our "Mary Kay" faces at all times. From the moment we awoke to the moment we hit the bed at night, we were to represent the business. This was because we were trying to sell good facial care and appearance.

In the medical setting you too will have to do a little bit of selling your self, at all times of the day. Wearing a nice shirt and slacks or something comparable can be very effective. Scrubs are great, but you should try to keep a change of clothing at work so that you can change, if you won't be in the angio suite all day. My experience has been that, even most patients respond well to the professional image of a doctor. Just about everyone wears scrubs today, even the housekeeping staff. Not that there is anything wrong with the housekeeping staff, but I just wouldn't want one of them putting a needle in me. If you must wear scrubs, make sure you have your name and credentials visible on the scrub top. I have my scrubs embroidered with my name and the credentials clearly visible. Get your self some white lab jackets with your name and credentials on them as well. Use these when you have scrubs on or over dress attire. Keep your self well groomed. It's easy to let your self go, when you work 70 hour weeks, but a good appearance shows you take care of yourself and you will take care of the patient just the same. Keeping this in mind, self weight management should be just as important. We have come a long way and having had a huge struggle with weight myself, I know this is not easy. I have made it my priority to take care of my entire self and hopefully give the appearance that I will do the same for my employer and my patients alike. It doesn't hurt that this also gives me a great sense of confidence.

As uneasy as this subject may be, I must address the use of Language. Since moving here from India years ago, I have struggled to get a better grasp of the English language. We as radiology professionals are good at the medical jargon that is used, but our language can use a little help. Speaking in a well managed tone and using correct grammar shows how professional we truly are. Using Basic English terms instead of slang or medical jargon when explaining procedures, is beneficial not only to the patient, but to us as well. You will have no doubt in your mind that they (the patient and /or family) have actually understood what you are trying to convey. Be thoughtful of the patient and their family members. Sometimes the family wants to know more than the patient. It is alright to answer all of their questions and make them feel at ease, with proper consent of course. Remember, if something goes wrong with the patient it is the family who will find faults. Try to prevent what you may have to manage later. At least this is my philosophy.

Professional circles and being a part of them is essential to any medical practice, especially radiology which relies on referrals from other medical practices. Be helpful to the radiologist while being professional and by introducing your self to the referring doctors who are in your sphere. If possible try to get your radiologist to introduce you to his colleagues and other physicians. Go out of your way to attend conferences that are held by some of the specialists. Begin to mingle with the physician assistants and nurse practitioners at these events, since most of the primary care medicine is being practiced by these individuals. Give them a chance to know that you care about their patients whether it is a specialty or not, and you too will get something in return. This is an opportunity to learn what you need to do to keep this doctor or provider happy. If you know this, you can help your business grow. The bottom line must show that you are a contributory entity in your practice. What better way to achieve this than to build a new bigger referring base and by keeping the existing one satisfied?

Treating your staff with respect is paramount to your well being at any institution. Having this in mind you must also set boundaries. The staff will expect you to buy them lunches or sponsor events and want to shoot the breeze with you as if you were one of them. It's great to have that relationship, but sometimes they might be trying to get privileged information from you. Try to be careful and make sure you do not divulge any proprietary information, which your radiologists may have trusted you with. If you want to buy them treats and lunches to get them to like you, this is wrong. Don't do it, it won't work for the long run. If your intensions are sincere, then try to keep it to your budget. You also don't want to over do it and do more than what the radiologists offer them. Your group is now your ally. You never thought, you would totally go to the other side, but some things are inevitable. It is difficult to have personal relationships with the staff, unless you are truly trusting of that person. I have a few select friends who are sincere, but I still keep a tight lip and display professionalism when it comes to discussing my practice.

You may also have to turn the other cheek, when they are talking about medicine and are convinced that their answer is the right one. Just let it go. You may know better and if it doesn't make a difference in patient management it's not doing any harm. If you really want to pursue the issue, offer a Continuing Medical Education (CME) class on the topic. When you back up your advice with references, your staff will not only believe you, but will give you much earned respect. On the other hand if you don't know something, just say so and offer to research it and get back to the staff. It is so easy to hurt people's feelings and you may not get a second chance to mend the situation. After studying about interpersonal relationships, I have found that only a few very secure people can take criticism of what they have known for a lifetime. You may know this from your own experience. Be kind and you will be rewarded with approval.

In conclusion, my own experience has been that to achieve a good status in the work environment and the medical community, professionalism and attitude play key roles. When you have a bad day at the office, you may want to re-evaluate your actions and arrive at your own reasonable explanations. I just try to remember that I am dealing with not only people, but a whole family, a situation or a culture. You never know what's going on in someone's life when you get into an argument with them. I try to look at the big picture and try to realize if this one situation is going to make a big difference in any major matter, and then deal with people on that global realization. You also have a choice on how you want to approach your career and your relationships with people.

C.

HOSPITAL CREDENTIALING AFTER YOU GRADUATE

I may have covered some of this in the previous chapters, but will give you the specifics here. Below you will find a list of documents which may help speed up your credentialing process in a hospital setting. Before you go to the staffing office, you can make some calls to that office and find out when the medical staffing committee meetings are held. You should also find out when the medical executive committee meeting is held. They are both usually once per month. If you are the first RPA at this facility, your file will first go to the medical executive committee for approval of the new position and then to the staffing committee to approve you as filling that position. Make some contacts with the surrounding hospitals to see if they have any RPAs or RAs, then you can use this as precedence for your hospital. Usually if you are the first one in the area, then just the concept of the RPA will go to the executive committee. They will approve the position and then one month later the staffing committee will approve you as the RPA/RA. Your radiologists need to know this if they don't, because they will have to lobby for you while you are in training. Some radiologists confuse the RPA/RA with the general PA position. It is a rude awakening when they discover otherwise. Here's what your check list for approaching the credentialing issue looks like.

1.   Have your affiliate agreement in hand

2.   Have a copy of your scope of practice for the RPA/RA

3.   Make sure you have medical liability insurance

4.   Have a copy of all of your credentials (ARRT, ACLS, BCLS, CBRPA, state License)

5.   Have 2 copies and an original of the filled out appropriate medical privileges application.

6.   Have your Radiologist and any others who will be supervising you sign the application.

7.   Have at least 3 letter of recommendation from the radiologists who have trained you.

8.   Get a letter of recommendation from your place of employment, if it is not the same radiology group.

9.   Have a log of all of your procedures documented and signed off by a radiologist

10. Have a documentation of your CMEs

11. You may even have to put together a form which looks similar to the hospital's own credentialing form, for the RPA. See next section on "how to put together a credentialing form"

The Credentialing process will take approximately 90 days and you should prepare for this, if you are changing jobs. Educate your new employer on this issue, because you will need to be sponsored by them as an employee, before you can start the credentialing process. You may even ask for temporary privileges while you wait for the real thing. Most hospitals have the ability to grant this. The main thing to remember during of this is to be very patient. You will hit snags and it will upset you, but you will persevere, just as I have.

D.
HOW TO PUT TOGETHER A CREDENTIALING FORM

Most of us radiology lifers were not born to write contracts and policies, but this is what we must do now. Putting together a privileges form is simple if you have some guidelines. I am happy to provide you with some. After having written several of them myself, I can tell you that they all have some common items. Focus on the list below and you will have no problems.

1. Get a copy of the privileges form for physician assistants and nurse anesthetists or practitioners, from the medical staffing office

2. Use this form as your guide, because people respond well to familiarity

3. If you do not have a form for the RPA, (there is one example on the CBRPA website), then follow the general guidelines I have provided below

    a. Heading should have the hospital name and Title

    b. A place for your name

    c. Limitations of the form

    d. General Statement

    e. Rules for granting privileges

    f. Requirement for the position(CME, number of procedures per year)

    g. Next you should have 3 categories to divide the procedures in terms of supervision.

4. Have a signature line for each person who will grant the privileges

5. Attach the general form to the existing application and this should work.

I have provided an example of one of the general forms I have used in the past. You may use this as is or you can change it to look like the one used at the particular facility you are covering. Remember, there is an example on www.cbrpa.org also. If you are using the form provided in this book, you will have to modify it to your liking. My recommendation is to create one your self using this one and the CBRPA form as a guide. You can store it in the computer and modify it to any other facility specifications. You can also make changes to the procedures and you can fill in the name of the facility etc… Good luck. If you need help, you may contact me. I may even start offering a service to help credential people in different facilities. It remains an idea at this time, waiting for the demand.

(Name of facility)
Delineation of Privileges
Radiology Practitioner Assistant (RPA)

APPLICANT'S <u>PRINTED</u> NAME	APPLICANT'S SIGNATURE /DATE

The allied health professional applying for privileges in this specialty will complete this delineation form. The applicant/re-applicant shall be designated the privileges he/she is requesting.

General Statement: Sponsored Radiology Practitioner Assistants (RPAs) will at all times practice as a part of the radiology care team under the medical direction of a Radiologist with full privileges in the (Name of facility) Health Care System.

It is the responsibility of each applicant/re-applicant to provide documentation of training and current competence in the privileges requested. Indicate the specific privileges you are requesting.

REQUIREMENTS

RPA's must fulfill these requirements listed below:

    a. Current licensure as a registered radiologic technologist in the state of (Name)
    b. Successful completion of and graduation from a radiology practitioner assistant
        Training approved by the Board of Radiology Practitioner Assistants
    c. Certification by the American Registry of Radiologic Technologists (ARRT)
    d. Certification by the Certification Board of Radiology Practitioner Assistants (CBRPA)
    e. Continuing education must be maintained in field of radiology practitioner assistant

CORE PRIVILEGES/CLASS I/available (15min by phone/45min to hospital):

Yes [ ]   No [ ]   Diagnostic Fluoroscopy
Yes [ ]   No [ ]   Fluoroscopy including injection of contrast into catheters, T-tube, fistulas for diagnostic
        purposes
Yes [ ]   No [ ]   Placement of enteric tubes
Yes [ ]   No [ ]   Setting protocols for exams
Yes [ ]   No [ ]   Ability to obtain additional films on an ordered exam
Yes [ ]   No [ ]   Ability to obtain follow up on post-procedural patients
Yes [ ]   No [ ]   Check list general radiology procedures (see attached)

CLASS II (Indirect): Those privileges which may be exercised after consultation with the responsible Radiologist (15min to hospital).

Yes [ ]   No [ ]   Breast needle localization
Yes [ ]   No [ ]   Lymphoscintigraphy injection
Yes [ ]   No [ ]   Paracentesis with Sonography
Yes [ ]   No [ ]   Thoracentesis with Sonography
Yes [ ]   No [ ]   Image guided Aspiration
Yes [ ]   No [ ]   Image guided PICC line placement
Yes [ ]   No [ ]   Image guided Lumbar puncture

CLASS III Privileges (Direct): Those privileges which may be exercised under the direct guidance or medical direction of the responsible Radiologist (Rad in Hospital).

Yes [ ]   No [ ]   Biopsy under CT/US guidance
Yes [ ]   No [ ]   Assisting radiologist in procedures where competence proved

I have reviewed this delineation of privileges and I attest to the fact that this applicant is capable of performing all the procedures requested.

Sponsoring Physician Signature	Date

Signature of Specialty Service Chief	Date

NOTES (EMPLOYMENT AND CREDENTIALING)

CHAPTER 6

INTERACTIONS WHICH WILL MOLD YOUR CAREER

Strategies to further your career
Pushing the boundaries/contributions
Networking-support organizations
Don't forget the Thank You

A.
STRATEGIES TO FURTHER YOUR CAREER

Not every RPA will get a good contract with a radiology group and have only the radiologists to answer to, thus you must know and cater to the people who can make the difference. Being proactive and having your goals clearly in your mind can help you to be very successful in everything. Throughout this book I have asked you to get to know your self and what you truly want. If you have exercised this in the manner you should have, there should be little doubt in what your goals consist of. After reading many books and having conversations with successful doctors and executives, I can tell you that if you do not have goals and the plans on how to achieve them you are doomed. Along with goal setting and careful planning comes the responsibility of execution which most certainly will entail building interpersonal relationships with the people around you.

Someone close to me gave me a book to read, which I eventually perused after much reluctance. I didn't want to read another book after years of going to school. But I can assure you that it was well worth the time and effort. I would recommend this book to anyone who has either wanted to get ahead, wanted to be noticed by the boss, or just wants to know how to get along with people who are not very friendly to say the least. Have you ever had a co-worker who hates you, no matter what you are doing or have done in the past? A boss who neglects you, no matter what great job you have done? Or maybe a friend who suddenly says, "I don't want to be your friend anymore, because you don't understand me"? Well, what does that mean? Am I a bad person, because I can't please everyone? Or Am I so very shortsighted and I should have known these problems were going to come up? Many people struggle with this not only in the workplace, but in their social circles as well. I can only talk about the changes this book has made in my way of thinking. After reading it yourself you may have your own conclusions. The book is titled, "The 7 habits of highly effective people" by: Stephen R. Covey. It retails for about $14 and is well worth the investment.

The book helped me to discover what my core principles were and how they would affect my daily activities and the way I viewed others. More importantly it helped me to decide if I was even driven by my principles alone, or were there other factors which drove my actions and reactions. Sometimes it's not what we know or care about, but the habits we have developed over time and our ability to change them if they become destructive. The author of the book defines habit as, "an intersection of knowledge, skill and desire". Maybe sometimes desire can get in the way of the other two or help utilize them more effectively? This has been my finding in the past. You too must decide if you can benefit from an exploration of your self and change your way of reaction.

Most people can act on an issue, but it is our reactions and the lack of control exhibited in those reactions which cause us the most grief. If you truly want to be the best of the best and get to the top, my suggestion is to get the book. I only wished that I had read it sooner. Well, it's never too late.

Aside from reading, life experiences offer the rest. The people you know and the impact you have on a situation can set the stage for good things to follow or disaster to loom over you just the same. Controlling the situation is not always an option or a possibility. For instance if you are performing fluoroscopy and you have been doing this for the last several months and now the management has asked a radiologist to ask you to teach a technologist to do your job. What will you do? Will you act in a proactive and decisive manner or will you just react with conviction to your beliefs as an angry child? You may not believe it, but I have seen the later in the workplace. This creates a very uncomfortable situation for the people who have trained you and may have paid for your schooling. I frankly don't know what a person should do in this situation, but when I was confronted with this, I had to do some research and make my own decisions. I looked at all sides of the scenario and made the pros and con list of issues surrounding the teaching issue. I tried not to make it personal. Instead, I tried to approach this in a business manner. What would happen if I trained the technologists and they missed pathology? Or what legal actions could be taken against me for instructing? How comfortable did I feel in instructing a technologist to perform procedures which involve a fair amount of didactic work as well as the hands on training? What monetary gains were on the table? If you look at all sides of a situation, you may find as I did, that you don't have to come across as a person who is taking it "personally". Keeping it out of the "personal" category is the key to preventing hard feelings and keeping the uncomfortable situations to a minimum. At least this has been my experience.

Attitude can be perceived from a distance. Having a good one can give you the edge that can make or break not only your day, but your whole career. I bowed out of a raise in salary and a chance to be a part of the executive team because of my beliefs as a RPA who did not want to train technologists to perform fluoroscopy. For my refusal, I stated the reasons as being legal and teaching related rather than personal ones. This gave me an out. Some administrators had their own ideas about why I did not want to take the task, but they had to respect my decision. The company later did decide to train their own fluoroscopy technologists and at this point I made a decision to seek employment elsewhere. If a radiology group does not see your potential and will not respect you for your training then there probably is not a good future in site, especially for you as an RPA or RA. Some people who have families and do not want to move would just stay on and keep their position, but this was not for me. I have discovered that most people are not "like" me. To generalize I would have to say most radiologic technologists I have met do work more than one job, do have the ambition, but like the "status quo" and if they step outside of their environment, they feel very insecure. This is just what I have seen. On the other hand the RPA students are quite the opposite and like to take on challenges and welcome change. In any case there are a few ideas I can share with you that seem to work for most.

The key aspect in any situations remains to be attitude, attitude, and attitude. Whether you are preparing for a job interview or just a meeting with the boss, you can utilize some or all of the ideas addressed here. Keeping a professional appearance is important most of the time. There are some times when you want to dress down a little so that you don't make the other person feel uncomfortable, especially if they are your boss. I would have to say hat if I was going for and interview; I would dress my best no matter what the scenario. The boss can look any way they want, but you have to look professional. So think about what you want to accomplish before you pick out your ensemble. Next you should be prepared for the meeting. Try to get a phone call with the person you are about to meet to find out what sorts of issues might come up. It is alright to ask, "Is there anything in particular I can prepare to discuss?" Or, "Would you like me to do any research on a matter before the meeting?" After you get your answers, don't forget to follow through and prepare for the issues in question. If you are unable to get any feedback before going into the meeting, then you can try the basics.

I try to make a list of all of my positive and negative contributions toward any given scenario. If I do this then I can have a good idea of what hurdles I will need to overcome during the meeting or an event. I have to think like the person who is opposite me. This way I can get a good idea of how they see me and what they are expecting from me. Hopefully you will not see just the negatives and scare yourselves right out of meeting the challenge. This is not what is meant by this exercise. I don't think you are of this sort of personality, because you are expanding your field, fighting battles and learning new medical tasks. Surely, you will have imagined the negative scenarios of a difficult biopsy before you decide to perform it. You may have also then tried to do the research to avoid the unnecessary risks and will watch for any other obstacles just the same. And so, when you do perform your first biopsy, you will try to make it a success. If you have planned for the worst and expected the best outcome, then you will have done all that may be asked of you, no matter what the result. This is all anyone can ask of a human being.

We tend to get in bad habits and forget the simple rules of the radiology profession. Rules like let the radiologists run the show and cater to the administrators, but don't forget to stand up for your self. Let them see that you are different and you are aware of your importance. You will still have to let the radiologists win a little, because after all they are the ones who took a chance on you as a radiologist extender and trained you to be who you are in their practice. Try to keep this in mind next time they are inconsiderate and grumpy. With the work load increasing and their revenue decreasing, they are extremely stressed. They tend to let the administrators run the company and their staff no matter what good intentions they may have for such staff. Being close with the administrators and supervisors will give you a chance for a fair battle when the situation arises. Most administrators are politicians. They have read all of the books and have attended seminars which teach them how to avoid conflict and manage situations. They can keep a poker face at almost any given situation. A gentle persuasion is what you might need to get close to one. Become a politician. Now there's an idea, I never thought I would approve let alone promote.

B.

Pushing the boundaries/contributions

When you have found your self in a comfortable place with regards to career, life and content-ment, thought should be given to giving back. Yes, giving back to the ones who can benefit from your experiences. I have tried to ask myself, "What can I give back to the people who have done for me or may benefit from my struggles?" Some of us are natural adventure seekers and the ones who like to push the boundaries and volunteer for just about anything. Just because you are not like "some of us", doesn't mean you can not contribute in your own way. I am sure many of you already do. Everyone has something to offer. Your experiences can be used to help so many others coming behind you.

People need to know that there are others out there with the same hurdles and problems that they themselves are facing. Not everyone can go out and help pass a law in their state for the RPA/RA occupation, but everyone can play a small part. My goal for the next year is to unite the RPAs/RAs who are living in Texas. I would like to form a group which will have an open forum where people can exchange ideas and learn to support each other. I know of others who have unit-ed some of their colleagues and challenged state laws. By far, I feel this is our biggest challenge. If we can focus as a group to devote even an hour a week out of our busy schedule to this cause, we can make a difference! Many RPAs don't even exchange words through the NSRPA web site chat room. I would like to see more traffic through that site. Who knows it may be therapeutic for you to just vent and let the rest of us know what is bothering you about the RPA world. Communica-tion is essential in any group think and I think we can be better about this.

Along with communication and the daring need to change laws, gaining our fair share of the job market is crucial. Many of us work along side other physician extenders who are not adequate-ly trained in radiology. There are efforts by the ASRT to have these persons get the much needed education in radiology. Their point is that they are trying to help promote better patient care by helping these professionals who are already in the radiology setting, but are lacking radiology specific education. You can be your own judge of this scenario, but many fear that this will open a door for more physician extenders outside of radiology to gain just enough radiology knowledge to be able to steal jobs away from the RPAs and the radiologist assistants. Keep abreast of this is-sue and if you come across it, try to understand it and form your own conclusions. We as a group can also have our voices heard if we have an opportunity to speak at a radiology conference or other forum.

Some of us in the RPA/RA pool are pretty good speakers. I have had the opportunity to hear many of them speaking out with conviction. It's true that this was merely at the NSRPA conference discussions and/or in front of other radiology professionals. My point is that maybe we should use our voices of conviction to speak to others besides the RPA community which already sympathizes with the RPAs. Take your convictions and instead of preaching to the choir, try preaching to radiologists, nurses, administrators, medical societies, and any one who will listen. We have to make our presence known and we have to do this quickly and consistently. At the last year's Radiologic Society of North America (RSNA) conference in 2003, I found that a hand full of people knew of the RPA concept. There was a lecture on how to use the RPA, NPs and PAs in radiology, but the person presenting had no knowledge of the RPA. I spent almost an hour after the lecture answering RPA related questions for the radiologists and radiology administrators. I have contacted the selection committee for the courses offered at the next RSNA about doing a lecture on the RPA/RA subject, but they have filled the slots for this year and are considering the talk for 2005. Even if I don't get a chance to speak out on this issue, at least I will have tried and this is all one can ask of someone. There is a definite disconnect between the radiologist community and the technologist community, and there exists a need for oral presentation and representation of and by the radiologist extender.

In June of 2004, I attended the ASRT conference in Dallas, Texas. I also decided to attend the educators' conference which preceded the technologist portion two days earlier. I found that there was in fact adequate talk about the RA at this meeting, but no radiologists in attendance! It just makes me think. Again we are telling a tale to the parties who are already in the know. Maybe, I am mistaken and everything will just take care of itself or then again maybe I am not. I think that we can make our own destiny and no matter how many procedures we can perform and how much time we can save the radiologists, until we market ourselves effectively, we are just under selling ourselves.

C.

NETWORKING-SUPPORT ORGANIZATIONS

You as the RPAs/RAs are very lucky to have a support structure in place. A place for guidance and support. When many new professions emerge, there is no one to steer you. We must thank the first few classes from Weber State University and Dr. Van Valkenburg for setting up a national society which is thriving. It is true that as a technologist we have the American Society for Radiologic Technologists (ASRT) and our local organizations, but the National Society for Radiology Practitioner Assistants (NSRPA) is unique to the RPA body.

The NSRPA membership has been growing and the members actually participate in making it better. The society welcomes the RAs as well as the radiology extenders from the 1970s. Your support in your own organization will mold your profession. You may have heard this before from some huge professional society, but it is so very true in this case. When the organization is young, you must make an impact and strive to grow the profession. You are trying to grow your practice at home and grow as a person, so why not grow the profession? It is a great feeling to help yet another RPA/RA to get out into the job market and succeed! You can find all of the information you need on their web site listed in Chapter 3. Member contact information, conferences, Job openings, RPA curriculum, RPA chat room, Legal matters, Billing and other helpful links are just some of the areas included.

The organization has an annual conference, usually held in Las Vegas, Nevada and features some of the most highly sought after speakers in radiology. These doctors support what we are doing and are happy to honor us at the conferences. You will have a chance to not only get valuable CMEs, but you may also attend a workshop for common procedures. You should make it a point to start saving early and not only join the NSRPA, but attend the meeting. There is a tremendous opportunity to network with your classmates and the practicing RPAs/RAs. In the future, there may be scholarships set up for people who just don't have the money to attend. Before you decide it is too expensive to attend, you should contact the person who will chair the conference or contact the NSRPA board. The NSRPA tries to choose dedicated and compassionate people to head any task committees. You will find that they will help you when you need them.

Some of the other organizations which are traditionally for the Radiologists are also important to join. The American Roentgen Ray Society (ARRS) has made a place for us, as a well as some of the other societies. Society for Interventional Radiology (SIR) has also welcomed us and is sending a representative to the NSRPA conference to show their support. Belonging to these societies sends a signal to the whole medical community that we are being accepted. We can learn about the issues that are important to them as physicians and also get a chance to network. When I was at the Radiological Society of North America (RSNA) last year, I was offered three RPA employment opportunities and many leads for a proposal presentation. Many physicians just do not know that we exist, let alone what we are capable of doing for their practice. It is an investment to attend these conferences and be a member in organizations, but ask any sales person. It is not the person who has the best product that makes the sale it is usually the person with a good product and a great marketing plan. If you add the networking and the people you know to the equation, the possibilities are endless for our growth. The choice is yours.

D.

DON'T FORGET THE THANK YOU

Well, none of us have gotten here alone, so it's only fitting that we thank the people who have helped us along the way. Sometimes it is difficult to send out cards, letters or e-mails thanking people who have meant so much to your career and your wellbeing, but it's never too late. Whether it's been a year or ten, the person who gets a sincere thank you will cherish it.

I am just as guilty as many of you may be. I have had good intentions of sending out appreciation gifts and cards yet fell short at times. Things just got in the way or I was working long hours. Maybe the family decided to come into town the weekend I was going to work on gift baskets. I can think of many hindrances to my plans and the time just ran away from me. So what am I doing differently now? Well, I decided to budget time into my project for that important task of writing personalized thank you notes and mailing them to the people who definitely deserve it. Most people will tell you that they didn't help you to get appreciation; they just did it to help you. Never the less, they will think very highly of you for remembering the little things in life that have a big impact. Don't you appreciate it when you get a thank you card from a relative after their visit to your home? You probably weren't expecting it or would have even cared if they didn't send you one in the first place, but when you do get it you do feel better about your self and how hospitable you must have been to deserve a card. I know I do. It's about making the person who helped you in your time of need feel a little better about them selves too. They may be having a bad day when they get your sweet note and this can have a positive impact. So try to think of what kind of an impact their advice or good gesture had on your life and appreciate them accordingly.

Who to thank? Make a list. This is an easy task. Maybe it's the file room person who holds interesting cases for you to look at and study, or a nurse who gives you heads up on a patient's condition when you are in a hurry. It's not just the doctors and the teachers, but some of the support staff, without whom you could not be where you are today. It is a way of life to be appreciative and to be appreciated in return. I guess I must have given enough praise to the file room staff at the trauma center where I trained, because I can still call in a favor when I need something. It's a way of life now. I just wish that I had done more for these staff members to let them know how much I did appreciate their support. Maybe they'll read this book and wonder if I am talking about them. I am.

All thanks aside, as a simple courtesy, people should do what's right. Most of traditional values have been getting away from us and some people think we are too pretentious for hanging on to them, but I never saw anything wrong with what goes on in the rest of the world. In India we greet our elders by bending at the knees and touching their feet. They may not even be related to us. Could you imagine an American doing this? Most of the world has not forgotten to give thanks to the people who have made their life of existence a possibility, let alone an enjoyable one. I hope I have convinced you to make time for this very important aspect of being a person, not only a professional.

NOTES (GETTING AHEAD IN YOUR CAREER)

CHAPTER 7
DOWN TO EARTH PRACTICES

Finding the right role
One success story after another

A.

Finding the right role

Graduation from the RPA/RA program and passing the CBRPA or ARRT examination is just the beginning of what can be a very prosperous and rewarding future. The RPA/RA of today has numerous possibilities for growth or stability. What ever they choose they can accomplish. A little inspiration never hurt anyone, so I am going to share some tasks I have been successful in achieving. Since graduating from RPA Program, I have had the opportunity to work with a radiology group performing exams and interpreting images under the radiologist's supervision. Even though I was successful at this, I still wanted to challenge myself further. So, I tried my hand at teaching, consulting and now writing. Whether I am a huge success or a little less, by trying I can test if something works for me or not.

Many of my friends are working in radiology groups performing procedures which are within the scope of practice for the RPA. They are putting in PICC lines, performing biopsies, placing drainage tubes, doing myelography, arthrography and other "ographies". They are also seeing patients before and after the invasive angiographic procedures and assisting the radiologists during those procedures. I have functioned as a sole fluoroscopist at times and then have function as a minor invasives radiologist, in the hospital setting. What ever your heart desires, there is a practice for you. You may have to move there to be in it, but it exists. Some RPAs are running entire clinics, because we make great liaisons between patients, radiologists, referring doctors and the support staff. To keep the peace, I feel we are the best management tool that exists today. We are however in a short supply and thus we can make the future we desire.

Did you realize that we as RPA/RAs are very good at radiology tasks and issues? Nothing you didn't realize your self, right? This may be a surprise to you, but you do have it within your self to not only entertain the idea of branching out, but to actually succeed! When I think of the RPA/RA, I think of a professional who has seen and captured an opportunity in the making. We didn't choose the path most traveled or the mainstream radiology trend. We chose to be different and try something that has a greater potential than conceived at this very moment. We as the RPA/RAs can either work for a radiologist doing their assigned tasks, or someone who may want to explore a little further! Many opportunities may be available to you, if you really want them, such as; managing a multimodality imaging center, Teaching, Consultation practice (Medical Legal, planning radiology practices, marketing new RPAs), Writing, and speaking at Conferences. The more we push ourselves, the more we can see ourselves accomplishing what we thought was impossible. Everyday, I think of new ways to utilize my new earned skills and knowledge base. You can truly be an independent person, being able to make your own destiny.

When my parents decided to immigrate to the United States, I came kicking and screaming. I asked my father repeatedly about the reasons for such a drastic move. Whenever I asked him about it, he would tell me it was to give us (the children) more opportunities. He further went on to say that being a girl, I would benefit more from the opportunities here in the states. Every time I get tired of doing something, I tell myself that a lot of sacrifices have been made to bring me to this land of opportunity and I must seize it every chance I get. Most of you have been born and raised here and maybe don't realize what comes so easily to you, but I am sure most of you soon will. I try to tell my self that when the occasion arises, you have to get out of your comfort zone and just do it! You as radiologic technologists and extenders have known radiology for a long time and you may have so many contributions yet to offer. Don't sell your self short.

I have been receiving at least two employment opportunities per month via e-mail, for graduating RPAs. This may mean moving to another place, but there are many more job prospects than there are RPAs to fill them. From physician extenders to directors of the educational programs, RPAs/RAs are in demand. The choice is always yours.

B.

ONE SUCCESS STORY AFTER ANOTHER

As you may have doubts about your RPA/RA roles, or even if you will succeed in the program, let me share this little story with you. One of my good friends, who asked me not to reveal any names, wanted you to have courage and remember that everyone has doubts. When you have doubts, read these stories and have courage.

"I remember being in x-ray school when I first heard about the RPA program at Weber State University in Utah. It caught my attention but since I was still in the beginning of my career, I dismissed the idea. However, I thought that it would be a great opportunity in the future.

When I graduated from the x-ray program, I wanted more than the role of a technologist. I pursued the career pathway of medical school. I went to Penn State University for a degree in biochemistry and a year in genetic research. When it came to the decision of medical school, I was undecided due to the requirements. I then remembered the RPA program. The role of the RPA was everything I was looking for. I enrolled at WSU and started my first semester. I was the only applicant to be involved in such a pioneer field from Pennsylvania. The first semester was brutal due to the heavy course load. However, the courses that we had I needed to do my job as an RPA. I remember spending late nights and all weekend studying and doing homework. I asked myself many times if this was worth the effort and risk. I remember feeling like nothing made sense as far as the criteria and how does all this fit together. I found out that there is a magical time in your education where things start to come together and make sense. I just had to be patient for that time.

The WSU RPA program was very intense. I have the chance to work with patients and be involved on the diagnostic and therapeutic side of radiology. The RPA program prepared me very well for all the education and hands on experience that I needed to do my job efficiently and accurately. I worked long hours at home studying while supporting a family. With the great support of my family and the radiology group, I accomplished my goal. Even though it takes time and dedication, if one would want to achieve such a goal, I'm living proof that you can successfully fulfill your dreams to further your education in the radiology field."

There are some radiology practices in California, Colorado, North Carolina, New York, Pennsylvania and Florida, who cannot get enough of the RPAs. All of these practices are proceeding with caution, but are still backing the RPAs and hopefully will back the RAs just the same. I had another friend who has been highlighted in many radiology journals and you may have had the pleasure of meeting him. Next, he shares his story.

I wanted to showcase James Abraham RPA, because I feel his story represents what most radiologist extenders are facing today. I would hope that his struggles and triumphs will help you through your journey as you grow in the field of radiology.

James has been in the interventional radiology arena for many years. As many others may have done, he not only worked with the radiology residents, but in fact had a very big hand in their training. While working in a teaching facility at the University of New Mexico, James finally took advantage of one of the annual offers he would receive each year from radiologists departing their fellowships to start new practices or join an existing one and build new services. James was always flattered, and this last offer meant a big move to Montana. This was not just a pat on the back from yet another radiologist he had worked with, but a chance to supervise, work 'hands on' with procedures, and help build an interventional service.

Immediately after making the move, James quickly realized that this may not be all that he had hoped. Montana state laws geared toward the radiologic technologists were very antiquated. On top of this, the nurses knew as much or more about the technologist scope of practice as the radiologic technologists themselves. James shared a story with me much like some of the others I have heard. James did something to help a patient in need by assisting a radiologist in completing a procedure which the doctor was not accustomed to doing before. This is what got the ball rolling. James was threatened by his superiors for misconduct even though the radiologist was in the room supervising, assisting, and most importantly, approving every aspect of the procedure. The whole incident was a surprise to the radiologists who were just simply shocked at the limitations of the RT license in the state of Montana. Well, all was not lost.

James was very disappointed at the whole situation and wondered if there was anything he could change. I think if you ask most of the RPAs they will tell you that they have been there too. This incident did lead James and the radiologists of Northwest Imaging to investigate other alternatives to fulfill the original purpose of bringing James to their facility. After some research, James applied and was later accepted in the RPA program at Weber State University. After one and a half years, James could finally do some of the things he was able to do in New Mexico, until of course; he was reported for practicing outside his RT scope of practice for the state of Montana. Unfortunately, this would not be the first; James was reported for investigation two more times within 4 weeks. The two latter allegations were submitted before James could present to the state his information, support, and validation for the first incident. Once James' information from the radiology group, the hospital, and Weber State University was submitted, the investigating board dropped all charges and stated the 'case closed indefinitely'. Finally he was allowed to function in the clinical agenda of what is stated in the RPA scope of practice. He graduated from the RPA program in 2002.

After speaking with James, I discovered that he is a very giving person who is working with others on changing and revising the laws for RPA/RAs in Montana. After some of these changes come to fruition he will be able to obtain hospital privileges, until then, his radiologists back him one hundred percent and he has a very successful career working and building the interventional service at his hospital in Montana. James was also featured in an Aunt Minnie web site article which highlighted his duties as an RPA.

James' advice to new RPA/RA students is "to work hard and keep going like you are running a marathon. Don't stop for a long break or you will find it difficult to catch up to the homework". He also emphasized one should buy a voice recognition program like Dragon Speak to help with RPA studies. James is an active participant in the NSRPA affaires and the IR conference symposia. He is always willing to lend a hand to anyone who may need his help. I feel very fortunate to be able to share his story with you.

NOTES (ANY ROLE MODELS AND CONTACTS)

NOTES (ANY ROLE MODELS AND CONTACTS)

CHAPTER 8
INCORPORATING A RADIOLOGIST EXTENDER IN YOUR PRACTICE

The Proposal
In the words of other Radiologists
Areas in which you can see the RPA/RA as a benefit

A.
THE PROPOSAL

Objective: To introduce and gain support for the idea of RPA/RA

Introduction: Radiologists have been invaluable and irreplaceable members of the medical community, due to their unique specialty. In fact their rising demands on that specialty have lead to overworked radiologists. Using a RPA/RA to perform the less complex procedures and using them as the radiologists' extension, we can all benefit.

Justification: Physicians Assistants have been used to cut down costs and increase productivity in the health care industry for many years. Physician extenders can spend more time with the patients at a lower financial cost. With the rising cost of healthcare and the pressures to keep them down, we have no other choice than to run our practices more efficiently. We must increase productivity without sacrificing service. Patients of today are consumers and feel they should be able to get the quality of care they deserve. This means that they demand more time with the radiologist when they get a service. When the radiologist should be focusing on the more complex and high dollar items, they are pulled away to speak with patients, answer protocol questions, or to perform other lower tasks. The end result is that in a nine hour day you are limited to bill for a low number of high dollar items or you are spending another two or three hours reading. The only way to increase productivity without increasing the number of hours in a workday is to increase the number of high dollar items that are billed for that day.

The latest in turf wars: I recently read an article in Diagnostic Imaging Online which was dated September 23, 2004 titled, "Urologists eye CT scanners as reimbursement drops". If you thought that the turf battles were coming to a halt, think again. This author states that "due to decrease in reimbursement for outpatient treatment of prostate cancer, some urologists have turned to CT scanning as a means to counter the shortfall."

Solution: To increase efficiency one must be open to new ideas. RPA/RA professionals are highly trained individuals with at least five years of radiology experience. You can utilize these professionals to build your practice to include seeing patients for imaging procedures, which is not possible currently. The school is very intense and the clinicals are done through the preceptor cite. There are outlined scenarios in the following pages for you to consider which may need extra fellowship training.

Trends: Radiologist extenders are employed in almost every state in America according to the statistics at from Weber State University. There are only a small number of states who do not have practicing extenders, but this may be due to the limitation on the programs being offered.

The idea of the extenders was brought forth in 1980s by the University of Texas. UT confirmed with their study, that radiologic technologists were just as capable of performing fluoroscopic exams as the radiology residents. In the 1970's the concept of the radiology PA failed due to the lack of need. Today there is a great need and a pool of applicants which are promoting the growth of educational programs. The ASRT, ACR and CBRPA along with other organizations will help this to be a profession in the main stream.

Liability: As a student the Weber State program provides the liability insurance for the student. After graduation, the student can choose from a variety of sources. I have my through the TMLT in Texas.

Costs: There is approximately $15,000 in costs to attend the RPA program at Weber state, other schools may vary. You can choose to pay for the applicant's fees in return for a two year commitment, or you can choose only to become a preceptor and later decide if you want them to work for you.

Due dates: Usually if the applicant does not have a preceptor by the Dec 1 due date, they are disqualified from the selection process.

There are many ways in which you can utilize the radiologist extender. Many radiologists are either on one extreme or the other. Some will let the extender do everything from fluoroscopy to biopsies unsupervised, and some will not even let them handle a question from the patient or technologist doing CT. It all depends on the kind of relationship which is developed between the radiologist and extender as well as the life experiences of the radiologist. All in all you can truly see the extenders being accepted by radiologists as a whole. It is just a matter of time before more radiology practices will want to add RPA/RA persons to their practices. It will make them more competitive without sacrificing patient care. It doesn't hurt to give something as fresh as this a try. You have nothing to loose, but the amount of work you will have to do in a day. If this sounds too good to be true, you can always call some of your fellow radiologists and the ACR for guidance. I hope you will keep an open mind.

If you decide that you are willing to hire a radiology extender, then let me commend you for seeing into the future and embracing it. Now that you have a RPA/RA on board try to keep a few things in mind.

1. Most RPA/RAs are contracted persons.

2. They should get a salary about one third of what the radiologists in your group make in a similar role.

3. The benefits offered to an RPA should be along the same lines as the other radiologists, but in smaller amounts. Benefits should also include; continuing medical education and book fund, time off for conferences and training.

4. The extender must maintain medical liability insurance and your radiologist carrier should have no problem adding them on to your policy.

5. Administratively the extender should be under the medical director, like another radiologist to whom the other radiologists answer.

6. Place training wheels on your extender, unless you yourself have trained them. Believe it or not all radiologists do things a little bit differently and you should allow the new hire to get used to your ways.

7. Know the scope of practice and keep the duties of the RPA/RA within that scope.

8. Seek legal counsel if you have any questions about limitations and liability. In most cases you will be using the "delegation of duties" portion of the Medical Practice Act.

9. Billing issues are getting updated frequently, so stay current. Medicare may give the extenders a way to bill for services, but this is not certain as of yet.

10. Keep a list of resources (included in this book) to consult including the RPA/RA. This is the one area in which I have seen the RPA underutilized. After all they should know all about their own profession.

If you remember that it's going to be a learning process for both parties the employer and the employee, things should workout just fine. With busy lifestyles of physicians, some times it is difficult to nurture the new position. I am proud to say that most RPAs that I know have thick skins and can hold their own. They fight for what they believe in and persevere. The physician assistants and nurse practitioners have been around for decades and the medical community relies on them to deliver quality healthcare. In a few more years the radiology community will begin to rely on the radiologist extenders just the same.

B.

IN THE WORDS OF OTHER RADIOLOGISTS

Here is what some of the radiologists are saying about the utilization of radiologist extenders.

"From a Radiologists perspective, the RPA position has successfully bridged the gap between Radiologist and Technologist. As exam volumes increase, reimbursement dwindles and well trained radiologists remain scarce, the RPA becomes a viable and cost effective means of increasing efficiency. But that is not all. Our experience has been one of enhanced income opportunities, improved patient satisfaction, and streamlined work flow; all the result of a single RPA."

As indicated above, there are four main benefits of RPA's to Radiologists.

First, as an interventional radiologist working in a community hospital, the ability to defer nearly all of the relatively routine procedures to an RPA allows me to concentrate on the more complicated cases and also assist in a significant amount of the routine film reading. With the addition of our RPA, I am able to do the work of at least 1 ½ Radiologists each day. In essence, an RPA can successfully perform a significant portion of the duties traditionally requiring a physician, allowing the Radiologist to perform more of the duties absolutely requiring a physician. We cover 8 small community hospitals with all images "piped in" to our central community hospital via PACS. We plan on adding 2 more RPA's in the next year to obviate the need of a radiologist performing GI procedures and arthrograms at our outlying facilities. This will result in a significant time savings to us in both travel time and time performing the procedures.

Second, there is a cost savings to the system. Despite RPA salaries being higher than RT salaries, every minute saved by the Radiologist can be translated into productive film reading or procedures. The cost benefit is significant. One need only ask any Radiologist how much it is worth to be 50% more productive. Who reaps the benefits of this cost savings is dependent on the type of practice. In our private practice setting, the Radiologists are the main financial beneficiaries.

Third, patient satisfaction is improved. Most Radiologists would agree that quality time with patients has declined as the constraints on our time have grown. Having a well trained individual contacting patients before and after procedures, thoroughly discussing their case, and obtaining consent has improved the patients experience in our institution. While a well trained nurse can also fulfill this function (particularly in the setting of a special procedures lab), I believe having an RPA spending time with the patient before, during and after the procedure is superior because fully ½ our exams or more are performed nearly autonomously by the RPA. The much vaunted continuity of care has been achieved and, quite simply, the patients are happier.

Finally, work flow is improved. Physicians are notorious for making patients, technologists and other ancillary staff wait. This is not due to lack of caring; but rather our attention being stretched several different directions at once. It is not uncommon to have 4 call reports, 2 physicians waiting for consults, a nurse from the floor on hold and an emergency in the ER awaiting your attention all at once. An RPA keeping the work flow going while the Radiologist "puts out fires" is a breath of fresh air in an otherwise congested work environment.

The success of any physician extender venture is dependent on the relationship. Trust based on quality performance of procedures by the RPA must be developed. This necessitates the RPA aspire to a level of excellence. On a personal note, James Abraham (see feature article) is our RPA and my right hand man. A testament to his importance in our practice is clearly apparent when he is on vacation. Many procedures are put on hold and the schedule is kept as light as possible. Upon his return, we sigh with relief and vow to never allow him to take another vacation.

In summary, the RPA is a welcome wave of the future in radiology. Certainly, its success will be gauged on its practitioners; in our experience, the future is assured. We have found the RPA to be more of a colleague to the radiologist, more of a mentor to the Radiology Technologist, more of a facilitator to the nurse, more of an expeditor to the schedulers; but most of all, more of a comforter to the patient.

Hugh B. Cecil
Board Certified Radiologist
9/17/03

"RPA's are fast becoming a reality in the current radiology practice environment. To date, our experience has been positive with regards to improvement in daily workload and efficiency. In our practice the improvement has been realized in the special procedures area where Mr. Abraham has been a high-end technologist for many years. The RPA training program has given him the opportunity to expand his skills and to perform various procedures, many of which were previously considered outside his "scope of practice" as a technologist.

As noted in "A Day in the Life", the amount of work required both prior to, and following, an interventional procedure is significant and affects patient care. In our case, the use of an RPA has been like adding half a radiologist position. This addition has greatly improved the general level of patient care where, in an understaffed, busy practice, inefficiencies can cause time losses. Furthermore, in today's electronic age of remote interpretation, an RPA may provide benefits through the performance of limited procedures remotely such as upper GI's, barium enemas, arthrograms, etc.

In regards to the potential negative impact of RPA's on a radiology practice, we have found none. The scope of practice being instituted at the state level and the exclusion of interpretation privileges has made James an important ally as opposed to a competitor. Overall, the RPA is welcomed in our practice and will have a positive impact on radiology in the future."

William R. Benedetto
Board Certified Radiologist

"In a typical 10-hour work day, a radiologist extender doubles the time the radiologist has for reading and interpreting images."

Radiologist
Montana

C.

AREAS IN WHICH YOU CAN SEE THE RPA/RA AS A BENEFIT

As with any new resource, there is always a period of experimentation and this surely evident with the RPAs and RAs. Many radiology groups are giving the extenders a chance, but still have doubts about how to utilize them efficiently. Many doubts of billing issues and Medicare rules of supervision have plagued the job market for RPA/RAs. I have dealt with this in the last three years and I am sure this will not stop anytime soon. With the RPA salaries increasing along with demand, many radiology groups are hiring them without having a clear picture. I was recently hired by a small radiology group in Dallas, with a chance for a partnership. Sounds great doesn't it? It is, but we are going through those issues of finding a good fit for us both. I have privileges at a hospital to perform a variety of invasive and non-invasive procedures, but with some supervision. This made me happy, thinking that this is a big step for a hospital to take in allowing a new profession to be accepted. My doctors on the other hand had a different idea and wanted me to be able to do almost everything on my own without any supervision. This is where cost benefit ratios come into question.

If you do not have enough work for one and a half radiologists at one facility, you may not benefit from an extender. You should however keep in mind that just because you don't have the work today, this may not be the story in six months. And just because Medicare won't allow us to bill for services at this very moment, that it won't be different in the future. Since you can't just find RPAs hanging around looking for jobs, you must act with foresight. I think this is why I was hired and I do believe that given the chance the radiology group will benefit greatly from my addition. We have increasing business demands which can benefit from a versatile person as me the RPA. Here are a few scenarios which I have presented.

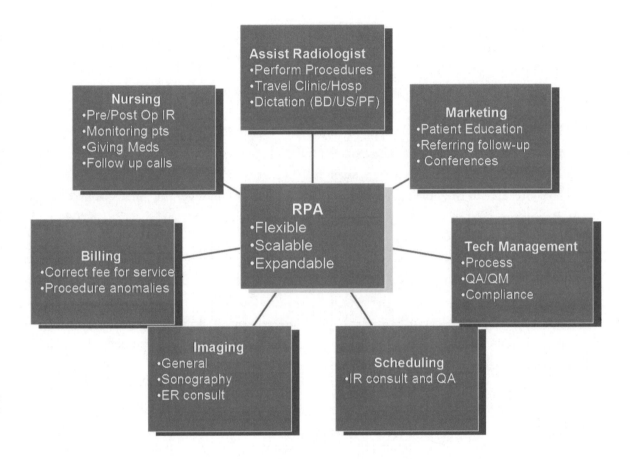

As the demand for mammography grows, discussion has begun on how to read the images in a more proficient manner. Radiologic Technology magazine September/October 2004 issue explains that physician extenders would be just the persons we need for such a task. Further, using programs in the U.K., an Institute of Medicine (IOM) report showed that studies of breast imaging practices in the U.K. indicate that trained non-physician healthcare professionals can interpret results with the same accuracy and speed as the radiologists. They stopped short of suggesting that non-radiologists could perform primary interpretations, but this report did suggest that mammography assistants could provide preliminary and or double-reading to aid Mammo-radiologist productivity. The above was taken from an article which also noted that there has been an 8.5% decrease in the number of facilities that provide mammography. The complete article, "ACR pans proposal to allow physician assistants to read mammography" dated 6/14/04 can be read on diagnostic imaging online.

Along with helping to fend of the decline in an imaging modality so cherished by its' patients and feared by the radiologists, the Radiologist Extenders trained in mammography can perform these double reads without the high rate of false positives which are evidently a problem with the Computer- Assisted Detection systems. Instead of CAD or in addition to it, consider the possibility of a RPA/RA. These extenders can also be a warm addition to your staff in helping the patient through a traumatic and fearful biopsy.

Another option for reading mammography is outsourcing, which is complicated due to international law and being too cost prohibitive for malpractice litigation. It is true that some of the imaging is being read by radiologist in other countries, but I just don't see this happening with mammography. There are too many guidelines and legal implications attached to this mater.

You can form your own opinions about the effective utilization of these mechanisms to promote better patient care in mammography. Having the ability to train your clone to help with mammography reading and diagnostic monitoring does have its advantages. No more will you have to argue over findings. You will have one person being trained by all of your partners and yourself to screen for cancerous suspects on the image. During my training, my radiologists actually enjoyed having me pre-screen the mammography images and point out any abnormalities. They told me that it broke the "monotony" and "a fresh pair of eyes", were always welcome.

One scenario that I myself presented to my preceptor is outlined on the next page.

Job Description for a mammography RPA position

- Works closely with radiologist to determine what is preferred in certain patient scenarios
- Acts as an extension of the Mammography radiologist as the first line of diagnostic imaging (spots and magnification views)
- Is able to obtain extra imaging to demonstrate the problematic area so that the imaging is complete and ready for reading by the radiologist
- Maybe the one who comforts an anxious patient who will be going through biopsy, other follow-up procedure or just wants a preliminary reading.
- Will assist with stereo-tactic biopsies and perform them after target confirmation by radiologist
- Act as a liaison between mammography and sonography technologists and the radiologist
- Be a patient advocate
- Preliminary or double reading with additional training

Benefits:

- Relieve overworked radiologist from remedial tasks
- Backlog of mammograms is decreased or eliminated
- Radiologist gets a second read and develops trust with RPA
- Radiologist can focus on surgical consults with specialists which helps to increase business

Qualifications:

- Mammography registered and fellowship trained RPA

Regulations:

- Radiologist must be on site for diagnostic mammography
- National and global efforts are underway to utilize physician extenders in this capacity
- ACR is in opposition to reading, but global studies show promise

Since radiologist extenders are being used commonly in a hospital setting, you may or may not need this diagram. I found this to be very helpful in presenting the RPA/RA to the radiologists. They in turn showed them to the "bean counters" and could get a better grasp of the cost vs. benefit ratio. After all radiologists are very visual people as we are. The scenario for the hospital setting may look like the diagram below:

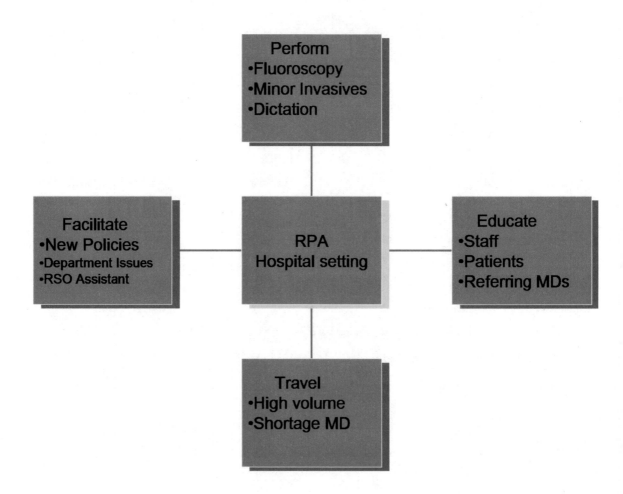

NOTES (WHAT TO TELL YOUR RADIOLOGISTS)

NOTES (WHAT TO TELL YOUR RADIOLOGISTS)

CHAPTER 9

DID I FORGET ANYTHING?

MISCELLANEOUS ITEMS WHICH MAY BE HELPFUL

1. When applying to the program, make sure you ask for your packet at least one to two months in advance (Sep/Oct)

2. Get recommendation letters from radiologists who would sponsor you

3. Have a preceptorship facility in mind and a back-up

4. Turn in the application to the program and the school by the end of November (due Dec 1st) for Weber, check for your school

5. When you go for orientation during the first visit to the University, go over all materials and make sure you have everything to do homework

6. Since you will be doing a distance learning model, you should look over the materials and be familiar with the rules

7. Make several copies of the homework face sheet. You may want to put your name and SS# on this before copying so that you do not have to keep writing this on the form

8. Go over the Modules or course materials and look at the first page and mark important due dates. Every teacher will be a little different, but this way you can make sure your work is being done in a timely manner.

9. You will do all of the major learning by doing tasks prompted at the beginning of the modules

10. You can either, e-mail, Fax, or snail mail your homework depending on the teacher. All of them will accept it via US Mail.

11. Collect interesting cases to present in class, which pertain to the area you are studying that semester.

12. Time at school should be spent doing school work and networking with other students

13. Invest in a Voice recognition software to help with homework

14. Make a list of all RPA/RAs in your state and keep their contact information by the phone... You will need it.

NOTES (YOUR SPECIFIC ISSUES AND HURDLES)

NOTES (YOUR SPECIFIC ISSUES AND HURDLES)

REFERENCES

Abella, H.A. (2003) Demand for techs soar, salaries follow. Diagnostic Imaging Online

Barnes, E. (2003) Hunting for recruits, pediatric radiologists take aim at "misconceptions". Auntminnie Online article

Brice, J (2004) IOM report urges use of physician extenders for preliminary mammography reads. Diagnostic Imaging Online

Brice, J. & Dakins, D.R. (2004) ACR, Institute of Medicine clash on technologists' role. Diagnostic Imaging Online

Brice, J. & Kaiser, C.P. (2004) ACR pans proposal to allow physician assistants to read mammography. Diagnostic Imaging Online

Brice, J. & Kaiser, C.P. (2004) Urologists eye CT scanners as reimbursement drops. Diagnostic Imaging Online

Burton, S.S. (2002) Radiology Practitioner Assistant. Advance for imaging and radiation therapy professionals. Vol. 15 (Issue 3) Page 20

Casey, B. (2003) RTs are already tackling advanced tasks, survey says. Auntminnie online article

Church, E.J. JD (2004) Legal Trends in Imaging. Radiologic Technology Vol.76.p.39

Covey, S.R. (1989) The 7 Habits of highly effective people. Fireside, New York.

De Gray, D. (2001) Are you burning out? Telltale Signs http://www.ivillage.com/topics/work/0,,165450,00.html

Farnsworth, L. (2002) Imaging by non-radiologists drives up healthcare costs. Auntminnie Online article

May, L. (2002) What is a Radiologist Assistant? Advance for Physician Assistants

Vining, D.J. MD (2003) The next Digital Frontier. Imaging Economics

Wolski, C (2004) *Staffing up. Imaging Economics*

General Web Sites used for research:

American Registry of Radiologic Technologists www.ARRT.org

American Society for Radiologic Technologists www.ASRT.org

Bloomsburg University www.bloomu.edu

Loma Linda University www.llu.edu

Massachusetts College of Pharmacy and Health Sciences www.mcp.edu

Midwestern State University www.mwsu.edu

Self help topics www.helpguide.org

Texas Sate Board of Nursing Examiners web site http://www.bne.state.tx.us/toc.htm

Texas State Board of Medical Examiners web site http://www.tsbme.state.tx.us/

University of Medicine and Dentistry at New Jersey www.umdnj.edu

University of North Carolina at Chapel Hill www.med.unc.edu

Weber State University www.Weber.edu

ISBN 1-41204697-1

9 781412 046978